Kinki Kreations

A PARENT'S GUIDE TO NATURAL BLACK HAIR CARE FOR KIDS

Jena Renee Williams

With Maida Cassandra Odom

HARLEM MOON
Broadway Books
New York

Published by Harlem Moon, an imprint of Broadway Books, a division of Random House, Inc.

PRINTED IN THE UNITED STATES OF AMERICA

HARLEM MOON, BROADWAY BOOKS, and the HARLEM MOON logo, depicting a moon and woman, are trademarks of Random House, Inc. The figure in the Harlem Moon logo is inspired by a graphic design by Aaron Douglas (1899–1979).

Visit our website at www.harlemmoon.com

Book design by Nicola Ferguson

Photo credits: Photos on pages 18, 28–30, 34, 51, 54, 55, 58, 64–71 copyright © Michelle Brooks; photos on pages 24, 25, 35–38, 42, 43, 49, 50, 52, 53, 56, 57, 59–62, 80, 81, 125, 126–133 copyright © Saundra Ali; photos on pages ii, 120, 121, 123, 134 copyright © Eric Von Lockhart; photos on pages 116, 117 copyright © Mateusz Krzesiczan; photos on pages 118, 119, 122 copyright © Elijah Lindsey.

Cataloging-in-Publication Data is on file with the Library of Congress.

ISBN 0-7679-1369-8

10 9 8 7 6 5 4 3 2

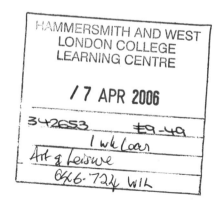

*This book is dedicated to all parents, my son Andre L. Rogers,
my future children, my godchildren, my little cousins, my
nieces and nephews, and colorful children all over the planet.*

A special thanks to the models
Taitianna
Imani Boniswa
Kadeem
Amir
Deione
Amber (Lady bug)
Chelsea
Tyra (Godiva)
Briana
Kiana
Toni
Melissa
Brandon
Chynna
Tykessa
Adia (Mooda)
Simone

Contents

Acknowledgments

This book's success is because of the support, growth, and development I've received from so many. I'll start off by thanking the Creator. I have to give a spiritual shout-out to the ancestors who paved a way for me, including my late great-grandmother (Grandmom Pinkie). I'd also like to thank my parents, Shirley and Charles Williams, my super supportive husband, Dwayne E. Rogers, and my amazing editor, Maida Odom.

Thank you to my agent Mike Bourret and Jane Dystel for taking a chance and supporting this book. Special thanks goes to my astonishing, brilliant, and patient editor, Clarence Haynes, and Janet Hill at Harlem Moon for truly believing in my book and making my dream come to life. Special thanks also to my Grandmom, Martha Holmes, my little brothers, Cornell Vanleer (Tony), Jomar Vanleer (Mar Mar), Carlton Brown (Puggy), my sister Julie Williams, and the staff at Kinki Kreations Braiding Salon. And additional thanks to my friends and team members, April Rose Battle, Clara Bell Singleton, Kim Rodgers, Caprice Troupe, Van Jackson, Terri Bracey, Adeyemi Kalenga, Brenda Thomas, Rachelle Ferrell (Queen Chelle), Queen Vemalaske, Kemp

David Satchel, Samia Cherry, Hakim Harrell (Cheezy), Norm Bond, my nieces Nashae Rogers and Amber Lathem (who volunteered lots of their teenage time to help me with photo shoots), Mister Mann Frisby, Karen Q. Miller, my spiritual mothers Barbara Daniels Cox, Lois Fernandez, Marjorie Vanleer, my teachers and mentors, Dr. Sonya Peterson Lewis, Sonia Sanchez, Kariamu Welsh Asante, Dr. Farrah Griffin, Diane Bailey, N'gone Sow Soween, Ademodela Mendella, Tulane Kinard, Cecilia Hinds, Ona Osirio-Matt, Gloria Johnson, William Roberts, Mr. Stanley Woods with the Goods, Faretta Spain, the parents of my beautiful models, and my beautiful models for their time and patience.

Kinki

Kreations

Testimony

About two years ago, a woman walked into my salon dragging a little girl behind her. She said she was there for a free consultation about her daughter's hair. As I looked at the woman, I could see from the expression on her face that she was tired. She said she was fed up and out of answers. Then I looked at her little girl. The child appeared to be afraid of the pain she thought she would encounter based on past experiences she'd had when her mother groomed her hair.

I walked over to the child and smiled. "Hello, pumpkin face," I said as I began examining her hair.

"Hi," she said shyly.

My cheery conversation hid my dismay. The little girl's hair and scalp were extremely damaged; what was left of her hair was battered, limp, and almost lifeless. From what I could see, her once healthy and full head of hair had been assaulted with chemical relaxers.

Her hair color was a dirty, dusty brown—probably a result of the chemical relaxers. Her hair texture was curly-tight at the roots, with a few straightened strands left on the ends. Her hair had been chopped off unevenly, patches of her scalp were burned and bald, and her hair ends were broken and split. I asked her mother what had happened.

"My daughter has nappy, untamable hair," her mother explained. "I'm tired of fighting with her every morning when it's time to have her hair combed for school. So I put a relaxer in it. And now look at it. Is there anything you can do?" she pleaded.

I cringed at her use of the word *nappy*. The girl's mother, like many parents of African-American children, was unable to see the beauty of her daughter's natural hair. Nor did she know how to nurture it because she lacked resources and a natural hair care background. Often parents take what they think is the easy way out, using a relaxer, but relaxers contain harsh chemicals that damage the hair and can affect the way children feel about their hair texture forever.

I asked the woman to have a seat.

Over the years, my skills, patience, creativity, and commitment had been put to the test, but never more so than with this sad little girl and her weary mother. Mentally and spiritually, I put on my gloves and green scrubs and prepared to perform an operation.

After shampooing the little girl's hair, I decided the best style for her would be small Senegalese twists gathered in a ponytail. I chose this style because it was low maintenance, light on her head, and it would cover the bald patches. I grabbed my shears, a wide-tooth comb, a rattail comb, synthetic hair, and my oil. Working carefully, I was able to create the illusion of fullness by adding a small amount of synthetic hair while also maintaining the child's youthful appearance with an age-appropriate style.

Once I was done, the mother and daughter looked at the new style in a mirror. The smiles on their faces were the inspiration for my children's salon and my decision to write this guide.

Healthy care for natural hair—that's what this book is all about.

Kinki Kreations provides instructions on how to care for the hair of Africans, African-Americans, Afro-Caribbeans, and all people who inherited their locks by way of the African Diaspora. This book also seeks to debunk myths and hopes to change attitudes about "good hair" versus "bad hair."

Kinki Kreations gives an overview of various hair textures and their roots, along with step-by-step grooming and styling directions. The styles and instructions offered cover the different age levels of children and the different skill levels of parents. Ten quick-and-easy styles are featured that showcase the beauty of natural hair.

Instructional photographs on styling and grooming are printed alongside the hair-care instructions. Braiding, twisting, shampooing, detangling hair, hair preparation, braid removal, and daily maintenance techniques are explained fully.

In addition to teaching grooming and styling, *Kinki Kreations* offers reliable reference materials and a glossary.

All over the world, people are exploring the glory of naturally kinky hair and wavy hair. Our beautiful, thick hair sometimes interlocks so tightly you can't get your fingers through it, let alone a comb. It is ours and we love it.

It is my hope that, after reading this book, more people will open their hearts, exhale, and join the legions of us who choose natural, healthy hair. Natural hair is a way of life, not a chore—that is my slogan, the slogan for my salon, and the message I'd like to emphasize to parents and caregivers.

Look at your son or daughter. Your child is also a child of the African Diaspora with the locks to prove it. It is my firm belief that hair grooming can be among your child's most enjoyable experiences after you learn the basics of proper hair care and the special properties of naturally kinky hair.

Kinki Kreations is dedicated to helping children celebrate their beautiful hair as they enjoy their beautiful lives. Children are our future and they are easily influenced. Tales of hair pulling and scalp burns during hair grooming are so common that they have become a mainstay of African-American literature and a traumatic part of our cultural experience. I'd like to change how parents and children feel about this intimate, important daily ritual.

The information in this book about self-love and taking care of kinky hair can serve as a powerful vehicle for African-American children on their trip to self-esteem and pride. This book can also be useful to adolescents as they grow into personal awareness and confidence.

There is great interest in natural hair these days. Natural hair stylists, like myself, have recognized that people are tired of the hair loss, broken edges, and split ends caused by chemicals. Some people who've been relaxing their hair for years are choosing healthy, natural hairstyles and enjoying the versatility that natural hair offers. Although many people want to wear their hair naturally, ignorance about natural hair care still abounds. Many permed, hot-curled African-American mothers, aunts, and grandmothers know nothing about natural hair care. This book will help many daughters, nieces, and granddaughters as they share and develop new grooming rituals.

Many African-American men are also caring for their children's hair these days, and this will be a valuable resource for brothers because most men are more familiar with the barbershop than with home hair-care rituals.

We also understand that a significant number of white parents and people of other races are adopting black children, taking in black foster children, and marrying into families with black children. (According to Ada White, director of Adoption Services at the Children's Welfare League of America, approximately 16 percent of adopted African-American children go to parents who are not of African-American descent.) These parents and caregivers are, understandably, lacking in the background, knowledge, and/or training necessary to ensure that their children's hair is properly groomed and maintained. Some nonblack caregivers attempt to groom a black child's hair the way they would groom their own, which can cause damage. *Kinki Kreations* will help them and the children in their care.

Kinki Kreations is for everyone who is interested in a better understanding of how to effectively and humanely care for kinky hair. For many, it will have the additional benefit of making them more comfortable with their own naturally textured hair.

It is my hope that salon owners, barbers, cosmetologists, and teachers will join parents in using this book and my carefully researched advice on maintaining "good hair" in all children to learn new skills and gain understanding. "Good hair," as I define it, is hair that is healthy and clean and not chemically altered.

Obviously, natural hair care is my passion. As a licensed stylist, braider, barber, and locktician, I've dedicated the last fourteen years of my life to studying hair and researching products. I've pioneered several new natural hair-care methods, braiding styles, and styling techniques such as the Casamas braid, an invisible stitch cornrow using kinky human hair and two-strand twists. I've mastered more than fifteen techniques in braiding, published three magazines on healthy hair care, and organized seminars on healthy hair care throughout the country. And at my natural hair-care salons, Kinki Kreations (for adults) and Kiddie Kreations (for children), I've regularly nurtured thousands of heads of hair back to health.

Please allow me to use my knowledge to take you and our kids higher.

Peace,

Jena Renée Williams

Introduction

Ask yourself a question:
If the stylist at a hair salon has to put on gloves to protect
her hands from the chemicals going onto your child's head,
then what do you think is happening to your baby's scalp?

Braiding is a form of art. It's one of the ways I freely express myself. I've been braiding hair since the age of five and been braiding professionally for fifteen years. I've braided, styled, and cared for thousands of heads of hair in my lifetime, taking care of hair textures ranging from curly-tight to straight and finding the style that best suits each person.

People constantly ask me, Why the obsession with natural hair? It began in 1987, during my sophomore year at Temple University in Philadelphia. I was the president of the African-American student union and was invited to attend a conference at Howard University in Washington, D.C., where the late Kwame Toure, formerly known as Stokely Carmichael, was the keynote speaker. Mr. Toure is best remembered as an outspoken militant civil rights leader who attacked racism all over the world. He was the chairman for the All-African People's Revolutionary Party (AARP), which worked toward ending the exploitation and subordination of black people.

While waiting for the lecture to begin, Toure and I were surrounded by a group of students like myself. There was a mixture of hairstyles among the crowd. I admired the braided hairstyle of one student. I complimented her and asked her how long she'd been wearing braids. We started debating the importance of natural hair. One sister shouted, "You can straighten your hair as long as you don't unbraid your mind."

Those words haunted me for a very long time. My choice then was to be a revolutionary-thinking person with my hair all fried-up. I was preaching and pushing natural hair care by encouraging black people to stop relaxing and straightening their hair, and yet I wasn't wearing my own hair in a natural style. As long as I stood by those words, I didn't have to be responsible for any of the suppressed hate I held for my own natural hair texture.

At the time, my hair was pressed with a straightening comb, or, as some folks call it, a hot comb. I'd been wearing my hair that way since high school. I was in full support of an African aesthetic, but I wouldn't be caught dead with natural hair because it honestly never occurred to me that wearing my own hair natural was an option if I wanted beauty, success, or love.

Secretly, I was afraid of natural hair. I thought that political activists like Angela Davis were doing a great job representing the aesthetics of natural black hair with their bountiful afros. They didn't need me.

When Kwame Toure began the lecture, he opened by acknowledging me. He mentioned that there was a powerful young sister in the audience who had great ideas and needed some direction. Toure spoke about the beauty of natural hair, and questioned why black folks hated their natural hair texture.

After the lecture, I began to question myself: Why did I choose relaxers? For me, hair straightening was part of a natural growing-up process, a rite of passage that just was supposed to happen.

My parents never believed in chemicals for my sister and me, not because they supported natural hair, but because my mom and dad believed my sister and I had "good hair." Our hair texture was wavy and easy to comb. When my hair was damp, with the aid of a little grease, my mother was able to style my hair into "pretty ponytails."

Other children used to ask me if I was mixed with white or Indian blood. I loved that question because it separated me from the "nappy-headed" kids. I felt that whatever mixed blood I had running through my veins saved me and my hair from the shame other children had to endure simply because of the texture of their hair.

I was beautiful in my own right, until my sister, Julie, was born. My sister's hair was straighter then mine. Julie's hair texture was like deeper waves in an ocean. Adults, as well as children, would compare my sister's hair texture to my hair texture and say, "Jena, your hair is pretty, but Julie's hair is prettier than yours. Jena, your hair is long but your sister's hair is longer." I heard this almost daily. At age five, it became clear to me that the straighter your hair was, the prettier you were considered to be and the more people liked you. I decided that since I didn't feel so beautiful anymore I would concentrate on excelling intellectually. I also started straightening my hair when I was fifteen.

Years later, when I was a freshman in college, hair still straightened, I was entering my apartment. A young brother walking by turned to me and said, "Hey, beautiful."

I looked around to see if he was talking to someone else because, up until then, only my parents and my grandmother had told me I was beautiful. I started to open my eyes to my own beauty, and the lecture by Brother Toure was the beginning of me embracing my natural hair.

Like the little girl who came into my salon with her mother, I was a victim of institutionalized racism. We'd adopted a beauty standard that was foreign to us by definition, but that was nonetheless passed on from generation to generation. Ultimately, this unhealthy way of thinking stems back to slavery, where we accepted the notion that our locks of hair were anything but beautiful because they didn't look like the oppressors'. We were not born hating our hair. It was taught to us.

Sometimes we relax our hair in the name of beauty, to be seen as beautiful by our brothers and sisters, or in an effort to fit into some white establishments. We seem to believe that as long as we don't remind white people that we are different, things will work well for us.

I eventually rejected that way of life. I became a recovering perm addict. I finally realized that generations of black folks have been and continue chemically destroying their hair and their children's hair.

I've been wearing my hair naturally for more than fifteen years now, around the same length of time I've been braiding hair professionally. I've worn cornrows, Casamas, individuals, Senegalese twists, two-strand twists, and flat twists, just to name a few. Natural is the only choice for me. It is my intention now to educate the minds and glorify the crowns of other kinky-headed folk in America.

With the support of Brother Toure and other friends, I published my first magazine, *Alternatives and Solutions*, in 1991. The magazine was filled with hairstyles and articles about natural hair care. Once the magazine was released, I felt a sense of accomplishment. I felt like I had offered solutions to all those who were in doubt about their natural hair. Now my strong love for black children has encouraged me to create this book, a parents' guide to children's needs.

The aesthetics and self-esteem of African-American children are in great jeopardy. Children continue to grow up believing that their kinky hair is not beautiful because of the implicit ignorance that is perpetuated through standards of beauty historically shown in magazines, television, and film and upheld by conversations between adults.

When someone speaks of nappy hair, usually they mean ugly, coarse, thick hair. It isn't mere chance that children as young as five years old know what nappy hair means. The constant conditioning and pressure from society forces children into believing that something is wrong with their hair, and thus with them.

This learned behavior encourages black children to crave anything that will make them "pretty" and their hair straight. But these children aren't knowledgeable about the chemicals in perms and relaxers or about the potential consequences of using them.

These products are damaging psychologically and physically. Straightening perpetuates the racist idea that a European standard of beauty is best. And alopecia, split ends, sores, and other scalp disorders are a few of the ill effects of chemical straightening. It hurts my heart to see the condition of a child's hair once some well-meaning parent has destroyed it with relaxers.

Healthy hair for children is vital. And natural hair is a way of life, not a fad. Parents must get "in touch" with their children's hair and learn to work with it. Once this happens, children will celebrate having their hair groomed.

I invite you to examine African hair as if for the first time. Allow yourself a fresh view of our beauty that has been ignored. This will enable you to understand a truly valid system of aesthetics that asserts itself without any apologies, independent of ignorance and prejudice.

Thankfully, natural hair has enjoyed a resurgence of popularity since the afros of the 1970s. I'm gratified when I look around and see how the number of African-American people wearing natural hairstyles has increased, particularly in my Philly neighborhood. Hats off to Erykah Badu, Lauryn Hill, Jill Scott, Alice Walker, Sonia Sanchez, Malcolm Jamal Warner, D'Angelo, Vanessa Williams, Allen Iverson, and all of the other athletes, entertainers, doctors, lawyers, and professionals who choose natural hair as a healthy alternative to the sad tradition and social conditioning that required self-deprecating hair straightening.

Although more people of African descent are choosing natural hairstyles, they still feel the pressures of internal racism. They still have to question themselves over their decision to be natural, and wonder if they'll still be considered attractive, or how it might affect their search for a job.

For black people, the way we choose to style our hair can factor into our professional success. There is little relationship between white people's hair texture and success—unless the hair is green, blue, purple, and spiked on top of their heads. I, and many others, would consider these chemically altered styles deviant. Yet black people's natural hair is considered deviant by many unless we change it to a looser, straighter texture.

But I stand firm in my belief that keeping it natural is what's best for our spirits. I love the process of bringing out my clients' natural beauty. Since 1998, I have been the proud owner of Kinki Kreations Braiding Salon. This salon specializes in natural, healthy hair care for African Americans. My highly trained staff of natural hair-care stylists and I take pride in our professionalism, customer service, and creativity. We realize that each client has different needs and offer more than forty hairstyle options.

In March 2000, I expanded my business and added a new salon exclusively for children between two and twelve years of age. Despite the growing numbers of us who've come to terms with our naturally kinky hair, there is an entire generation of children who are victims of overprocessed and damaged hair.

After doing a good job and making children happy, our main objective is to reeducate parents about healthy hair care for children. I'm very proud to have a salon that caters to both adults and the children in the same space, with each respective salon separated by banks of shampoo sinks and dryers. It's a one-stop shop. You and your child can be serviced at the same time and the salon is set up to be child friendly, so you don't have to worry about your child being bored and rushing you along. Making the hair-care experience enjoyable for children is one of my personal goals and is a goal of this book.

Another major goal of *Kinki Kreations* is to make your child's hair healthier, prettier, and better. Thoroughly combing hair, twisting, braiding, locking, unbraiding, and shampooing may seem to be a little difficult at first, but practice makes perfect. Parents must set the example by loving their children's natural hair so that natural hairstyling will continue and extend through generations. If you read *Kinki Kreations* in its entirety, you will find the help and answers you need.

1 A Note to Parents

I was a young child when I learned the difference between what people call "good" and "bad" hair.

The straighter your hair was, the more you were liked, and the prettier you were thought to be. That was "good hair." If your hair was tightly curled or kinky, you had "bad hair" and were considered less attractive.

I remember jumping double Dutch with some of my friends. A tall caramel-complexioned woman dressed in a black suit and white sneakers and carrying a briefcase walked by. She went over to my friend Tara, whose hair was styled in two long straight ponytails (pressed hard by a hot comb), and said, "Your hair is beautiful and soft." The woman then looked at me and my sister and said, "Oh my God, your hair is pretty also. Are you two twins? You girls have good hair. It's beautiful." The woman told us to be good girls and walked off.

She never said anything about Sheena's hair. Sheena's hair was short and tight. Her mother used to style her hair in tiny braids and connect them all going to the back. After the woman left, we teased Sheena. "Ah ha! That lady ain't say nothing about your nappy ugly stuff, and you're black and ugly, burnt like toast," someone said. We all sang the "you got nappy hair" song. Sheena got angry, took her jump rope, and ran into the house crying.

I was an adult before I truly understood how sad and hurtful that must have been for Sheena. Those hateful impressions and expressions can affect how others perceive that child and leave that child emotionally traumatized, even into adulthood.

For generations, African-American children have been victims of child abuse. They have been told over and over again that their hair is unmanageable, worthless, and ugly. In short, bad. This has been reinforced by television and film images, and also by marketers of hair straighteners. Sadly, the first application of a hair-straightening relaxer to a child's hair is synonymous with a "rite of passage" for some parents and their daughters. A first "perm," sadly, is seen as the beginning of adulthood, success, and social development.

According to manufacturer's instructions, gloves are required when applying any sort of chemical to hair. Think about the delicate scalp of your child, and then consider why you would slather it with chemicals too harsh for your own hands. Can you imagine what happens when the chemicals are allowed to sink into the pores of your child's tender scalp?

Obviously, these chemicals are dangerous; they can cause hair breakage, scalp sores, and bald patches.

Please, keep the chemicals out of your child's hair. Remember that texture and length are no mistake. Every person's hair length varies. One person's hair might only grow as long as an inch and stop, while others will grow 15 inches or longer over time. Don't get caught up in the length of a child's hair. Work the length as it is. Learn to be creative with whatever head of hair your child has, whatever you have to work with. Your acceptance of your child's natural attributes will help his or her self-esteem.

If your child has a perm, as you will learn in Chapter 9, there will be several challenges to getting the chemicals out. Perms must be cut off or allowed to grow out through gradual trimming. However, there are hairstyles to make this phase less awkward, which are also highlighted in Chapter 9.

Communicate to your children, as early as possible, the importance of natural healthy hair and how to appreciate its unique, special qualities. Refrain from using negative words to describe their hair like *nappy, peazy, hard-to-comb, untamable,* and any other word or phrase that could negatively affect a child's self-esteem.

Keeping Your Child's Crown Clean

Also talk to your child about not letting all sorts of hands in her hair. Have you ever experienced sending your child to school or the sitter with one hairstyle, only to have her come back home with a different one? Children like to experiment with one another's hair. Explain to your children that it isn't good to allow several hands in their hair. Children also tend to share the same comb and ornaments, which can cause the spread of scalp conditions and diseases such as tinea and alopecia.

If you do trust a sitter or a friend to care for your child's hair, then send your own bucket of hair tools along. Each child should have his or her own personal grooming tools. A list of these hair-grooming necessities is offered in Chapter 2. Having one's own personal implements cuts down on germs and the transmission of contagious diseases, a subject discussed more thoroughly in Chapter 17. (By the way, stay away from rubber bands. They're extremely damaging to the hair and cause breakage. Hair ornaments that are covered with cloth are wonderful alternatives. Hair tools and ornaments are discussed in more detail in Chapters 2 and 12.)

Sanitation is extremely important. It's very necessary to keep all implements and ornaments clean from dirt and debris. Using soap and hot water will kill most germs. Spray all hair-care and grooming implements with 70 percent alcohol. It's important to remember that "good hair" is hair that is healthy and clean.

Please also understand that healthy hair starts with a healthy diet. There is no mysterious formula. Drinking plenty of water and eating fresh fruits and vegetables are the components of a balanced diet that will assist in the nourishment of healthy skin and hair. Keep your child away from processed foods, fatty foods, and foods that contain lots of sugar. Good health starts from the inside out and healthy hair begins with your child's eating habits.

2 Getting Started—
Using the Proper Tools

Every parent should have a tool bucket that contains the vital implements and ornaments needed to style their child's hair. These tools can be purchased at any beauty supply store.

* ✳ RATTAIL COMB—great for making straight parts and removing debris from the hair.
* ✳ BRUSH (soft or medium boar bristles)—helps smooth hair.
* ✳ OIL—good for shine and provides some nutrients. Use oils that contain sage, olive, rosemary, and almond or lavender, which are great for the hair and scalp. Light oils in liquid, not gel, form are best.
* ✳ SPRAY BOTTLE—keep filled with one part oil and six parts water.
* ✳ BLOW DRYER—for quick drying and detangling.
* ✳ HAIR ORNAMENTS—bows, ribbon, barrettes, cloth-covered rubber bands (these will not break your child's hair), beads, ballies.
* ✳ HAIR PINS—assist in holding some styles securely.
* ✳ HAIR CLIPS—hold hair in place while styling.

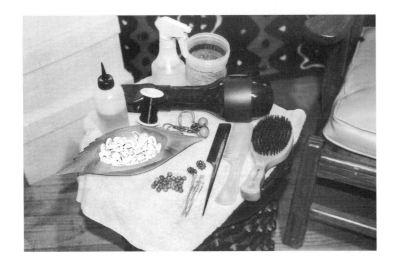

* PICK—wide teeth allow for combing through thick hair.
* WIDE-TOOTH COMB—helps detangle thick hair during a comb out.
* GEL—helps in styling and luster.
* SHAMPOO AND CONDITIONER—Aveda, Carol's Daughter, Praises, and Organic Root Stimulator have also has some excellent products. You can generally find great natural shampoos and conditioners at natural health food stores.
* VIDEOTAPE OR DVD—for children to watch while sitting.

3 Child Profile Card

This can be a great way for you to monitor changes in the condition of your child's scalp and hair. This evaluation also will help you discover how well you understand your child's hair. Answer all of the questions as honestly as you can. You should also feel free to adjust the information we've provided on this form to meet your child's needs.

Before you begin filling the form out, examine your child's hair by separating sections of the hair at the base of the scalp. Look for any possible damage. You will be looking for areas where the hair is broken and/or thin while keeping an eye out for bald spots. Examine the hairline as well. Styles like cornrows and small braids can cause severe hair damage when certain problems, such as receding hairlines and balding edges, are present.

You will also be looking for cuts, sores, and scabs. If you find anything, write it down in the notes section of your profile card. These are the areas you will constantly monitor for the next twelve weeks.

Whenever your child is prescribed any medication, write down the dates he or she started and completed the medicine. Ask the doctor if there are any side effects. If you notice a change in your child's skin or hair, consult the doctor immediately and be sure to make a note of any changes for your own personal records.

Child Profile Card

1. Scalp condition	normal ❑	oily ❑	dry ❑
2. Hair condition	normal ❑	oily ❑	dry ❑
3. Hair density	thin ❑	medium ❑	thick ❑
4. Hair texture	straight ❑	wavy ❑	curly ❑
	tight curl ❑	very tight curl ❑	

1. List any medications and their side effects.

_____
_____
_____
_____

2. Any hair breakage?　　no ❑　　　　yes ❑ (explain why)

_____
_____
_____

3. Date of last trim (hair should be trimmed two to three times a year).

_____

4. List any scalp disorders.

_____
_____
_____
_____

4 What Is Hair?

The primary function of hair is to protect and insulate the body from the weather and to protect the head from injury. It also provides beauty and adornment.

The hair is divided into two parts; the hair **root** and the hair **shaft**. The hair root is the structure beneath the skin surface. The hair shaft extends above the skin surface.

The structure of the hair root is composed of three parts: the **follicle, bulb,** and **papilla.**

The follicle is composed of hydrogen, oxygen, carbon, sulfur, and phosphorus.

The bulb is a round structure at the very bottom of the hair root.

The papilla, which fits inside of the bulb, lies deep within the epidermis, nerves, and blood vessels. If you're in good health and take care of your body, maintaining a healthy diet (water, fruits, vegetables, fiber, etc.), the bulb will be nourished, thereby nourishing the papilla. The papilla is filled with a rich supply of nerves and blood, which contribute to the growth and regeneration of hair. As long as the papilla is well-nourished, it will provide healthy, natural hair that will grow.

A healthy hair root will also provide a healthy hair shaft. The structure of the hair shaft consists of three parts: the inner core, also known as the **medulla** (some hair types do not contain a medulla); the middle layer, which is the **cortex;** and the outer layer, which is the **cuticle.** The cortex is responsible for the strength, color, and texture of the hair, while the cuticle's main function is to protect the cortex.

If you use harsh chemicals, like relaxers, or you use a hot comb and/or excessive heat on the hair, you're affecting the growth and natural development of the cuticle. If the cuticle is badly damaged or destroyed, the cortex will be left unprotected, which leads to hair breakage that can go all the way down the hair shaft to the roots. Keeping your hair natural is the healthiest option.

5 Babies

Infants require special, but simple, hair care.

First of all, every baby's head has a soft spot at the top of the head called a fontanel. This spot should be handled with care. As the skull grows, the fontanel will eventually become firmer and disappear.

Some babies are born with lots of hair, while other babies are born with very little hair. Whether your baby has lots of hair or very little, your baby's scalp is fragile and the hair follicles are still developing, so your baby's hair and scalp need gentle care.

Parents tend to treat their newborns like dolls. This is fine, but when it comes to grooming your baby's hair, be careful. Don't pull the hair too tightly. And don't try to force styles that can't be accomplished with your child's hair because it's too short or too soft.

Please don't use rubber bands or hair ornaments that could easily come out of your baby's hair and find their way into his or her mouth. We all know how children like to put things in their mouths, and many hair ornaments are of a size that could cause choking, as well as being not particularly sanitary.

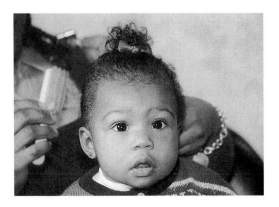

Help your family love and celebrate your baby's appearance whether your baby's hair is short, medium, or long.

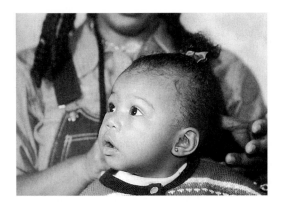

Keep your baby's hair covered with warm hats made with a soft crochet that is appropriate for the weather conditions. Babies' heads need to be protected from all types of weather, since they are particularly sensitive to the sun, heat, and cold.

You can clean your baby's hair and scalp with a washcloth and a natural, mild baby shampoo. Rinse the hair with lukewarm water, being careful not to get the soap in the baby's eyes. Rub a little oil on the hair and use a soft-bristle baby brush. Brush the baby's hair in the direction that it naturally grows. Very little maintenance is required.

After a few months, the baby's hair texture will begin to change. This is a normal process. Don't force the hair to do what you want it to do. Allow the hair to grow in naturally.

Some babies' hair grows faster. (Our hair's growth rate is determined by our genes.) Be patient.

Often a baby's hair will grow on the top while remaining thin on the sides and back of the scalp. This is normal. Baby's neck muscles are still developing and the baby's hair on both sides rubs off on bed linen and clothes. Eventually, your baby's hair will grow in all over.

Cradle cap, a type of dermatitis that appears as a crusty white or yellow patch on the scalp, is a common scalp condition found in babies. Cradle cap can look like patches of dandruff or a scabby white or yellowish substance forming on the scalp. Cradle cap is not dangerous. It usually goes away after the first year, but this could mean that your child could be prone to eczema. Don't scratch the surface of the baby's scalp, since this could cause irritation.

To treat cradle cap, simply use olive oil or baby oil to loosen the flakes, and then shampoo. If the cradle cap appears to be spreading across the scalp, face, and neck, or if there are signs of infection, consult a physician immediately.

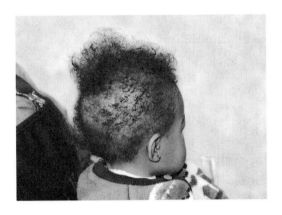

Often a baby's hair will grow on top while remaining thin on the sides and back of the scalp.

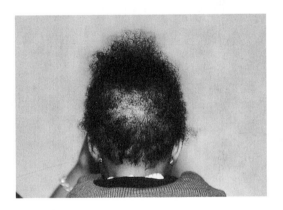

6 Shampooing

You should shampoo your child's hair every two weeks. Regular shampooing is important to remove dirt, debris, and oil residue, but shampooing too often can cause the hair to become dry and break off.

It helps to comb the hair through thoroughly before you shampoo your child's hair. This will prevent tangles and matting from forming.

The best, most effective, and comfortable way to shampoo your child's hair is by using a shampoo bowl. Unfortunately, most parents don't have shampoo bowls in their homes. So it's back to the old-fashioned way: having your child bend over the kitchen sink or under the bathroom tub faucet. Children two years of age and older can be held over the sink with assistance, while younger children can have their hair shampooed while taking a bath.

You may want to attach a removable spray nozzle to the sink or showerhead for shampooing your child's hair. A spray nozzle is a huge help in rinsing all of the soap out of your child's hair with a minimum of fuss.

Conditioning the hair is as important as shampooing the hair. Conditioners moisturize, soften, and detangle hair.

Here are the steps to effective shampooing:

1. Help your child kneel securely on a chair and lean over the sink.
2. Saturate the hair with water.
3. Squeeze some shampoo (about the circumference of a quarter) into the palm of your hand and gently massage the shampoo all over your child's hair. Estimate the amount of shampoo based on hair length. (You can never use too much shampoo as long as you rinse it out fully during the rinse.)
4. Using the ball of your fingertips (don't use your nails—scratching can irritate the scalp), massage the scalp and move your fingers through the hair starting around the hairline and the nape of the neck and working your way to the center of the scalp. Work effectively and quickly. Children tend to become uncomfortable if they are bent over the sink too long. Gently work the shampoo evenly throughout the hair.

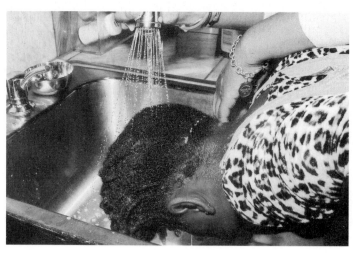

Step #2.

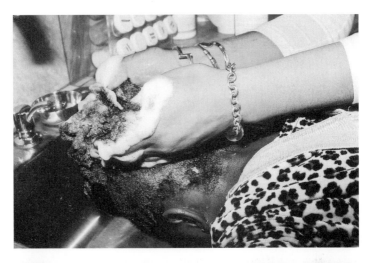

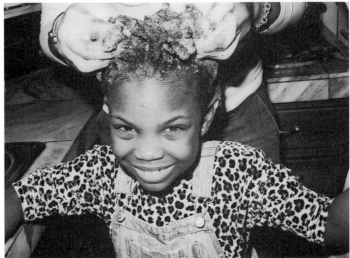

Step #4.

(Usually the first shampoo doesn't lather up that well, but keep in mind the detergent in the shampoo is, in fact, working.)

5. Rinse the hair thoroughly with warm water, making sure the hair is free of soapsuds. The water should run clear.

6. Repeat steps 2 through 4.

29

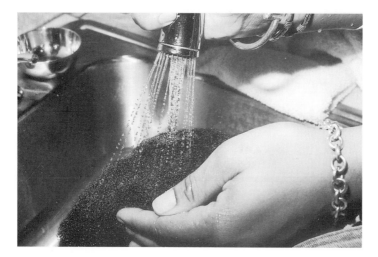

Step #5.

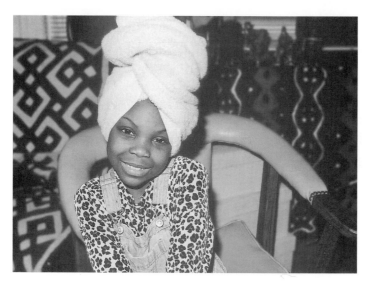

Step #10.

7. After all the shampoo is out, gently squeeze all the excess water from the hair.

8. Add about a handful of conditioner to your palm. Massage the conditioner all over the hair and allow it to sit on the hair for from 5 to 15 minutes.

9. Repeat steps 4, 5, and 7.

10. Gently towel dry.

Now we're ready for hair preparation!

7 Hair Preparation

Hair preparation is extremely important when styling hair. When the hair is properly cleaned, combed through, and oiled, styling can be a snap!

Before you start to style your child's hair, you will need tools from your tool bucket, discussed in Chapter 2.

* Your child's favorite book or video
* Large clips (clips need to be big enough to keep large sections of hair out of the way)
* Oil
* Ornaments
* A rattail comb
* A wide-tooth comb
* A boar-bristle brush
* A water bottle filled with six parts water and one part oil

Comb through

Using your rattail comb, part the hair into four to eight even sections. Gently separate the hair for comb through, using your fingers. The tighter the curl pattern of the hair, the more sections you'll need. The looser the curl pattern, the fewer sections are needed.

When using the rattail comb to part the hair into workable sections, it's not necessary to dig the comb into the scalp. This can cause irritation. If the hair appears to be tangled, gently pull the strands apart with your fingers. Be careful not to roughly rip the hair apart. Take your time so that you don't cause any pain to your child or damage to the hair.

After each section is separated, hold that section of hair together with a cloth-covered elastic band, or twist the section and hold it securely with a clip large enough to hold the section.

Remember the hair is still not combed through; we have just sectioned the

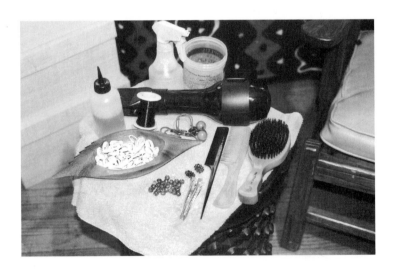

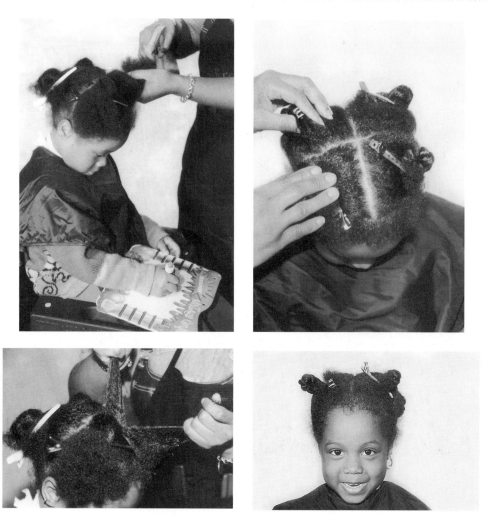

To prepare for comb through, after separating each section of hair, you can twist the section and hold it securely with a large clip.

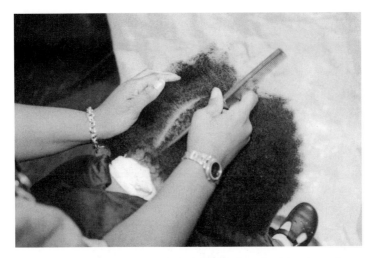

Unclip a section of hair and hold it firmly before combing through.

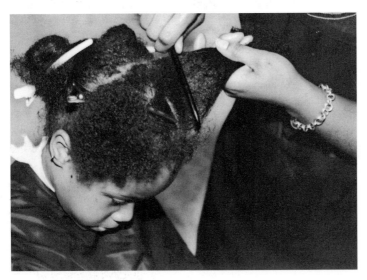

Using a wide-tooth comb, start combing the hair at the ends, working your way to the roots.

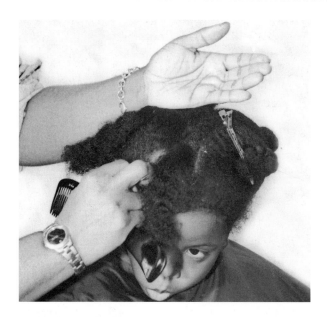

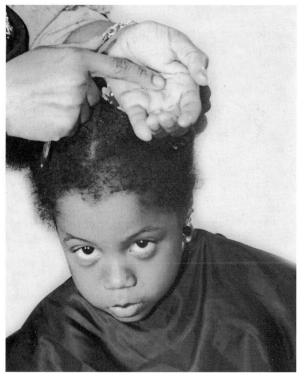

Apply hair oils that contain sage, olive, rosemary, almond, or lavender to the scalp.

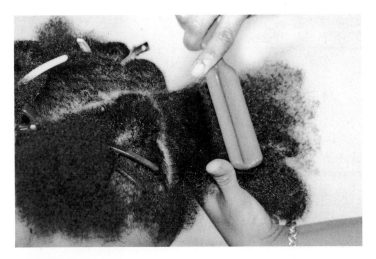

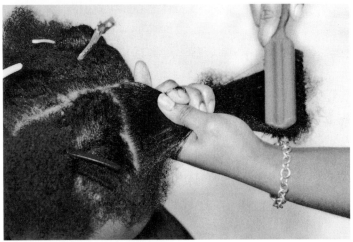

Using a boar-bristle brush, brush oil into the hair and then twist or braid each section so that it doesn't become tangled.

hair off so that we can begin the comb-through process, proceeding one section at a time.

Even if you've just finished a shampoo, it is important to have a spray bottle on hand. Sometimes hair tends to air-dry quickly, so after you comb through each section, add oil and water from your spray bottle and then brush hair to distribute the water-oil mixture. Because natural hair can tangle quickly, spraying the hair with a mixture of six parts water and one part oil will make the hair easier to comb through.

Once all the hair is sectioned, you are ready to comb the hair through. Starting from the nape of the neck, untwist or unclip a section of hair. Hold the hair firmly.

Using your wide-tooth comb, start combing the hair at the ends and work your way up to the roots. The movement should be quick but not painful to the child.

If your child complains about pain, listen and be gentle. Holding the hair by the root as you're combing through a section can prevent harsh pulling and pain. This will help you continue a good relationship with your child and make hair-grooming time pleasurable for both of you. Continue the described process until the section is fully combed through.

After all the hair is combed through, apply a small amount of oil to the scalp, making sure not to oversaturate the scalp, and massage a little oil all over the hair.

Use oils that contain sage, olive, rosemary, and almond or lavender, which are the best oils for the hair and scalp. Carol's Daughter and Praises provide excellent oils. Light oils that are in liquid form are best.

Avoid using heavy substances such as lanolin, petroleum, and mineral oils, since they attract dust and dirt and may clog the pores. If pores aren't able to breathe, this can slow the natural hair-growth process.

Using your boar-bristle brush, brush the oil into the hair, then twist and clip or braid each brushed section so that it doesn't become tangled as you work on the next section. Continue oiling and brushing until all the hair has been cared for.

Don't be alarmed by hair loss. We shed approximately one hundred strands of hair per day. It's normal to see a bundle of hair in the comb or brush at the end of post-shampoo hair preparation.

Blow-drying

Blow-drying the hair will make the hair straighter and easier to comb and style. Blow-dry the hair to assist in styling. This is a good alternative if you want to achieve a straighter look using harsh chemicals than can affect the scalp. But remember, too much heat of any kind, including a blow-dryer's, can be damaging.

After combing the hair through in hair preparation, unbraid or remove the clips from the separated sections and comb the hair all the way through again. Using the comb attachment of the blow-dryer, comb the hair, starting at the ends of the hair and working your way up to the root. Clip each section as you are finished.

Trimming Split Ends

Everyone gets split ends; they're almost impossible to escape. A split end occurs when a single strand of hair splits into two strands. The splitting of the strand causes the hair to become weak and brittle. Split ends are often caused by excessive blow drying, using incorrect tools to style the hair, and hair straightening with a hot comb, hot curlers, relaxers, or texturizers.

Using a pair of scissors made especially for hair will assist you in trimming the split ends of the hair. Giving your child a full haircut is not recommended. If your child needs a haircut, then I would suggest going to a professional.

You should trim the hair after blow-drying. Using your index or pointer finger as a guide, trim a length that is about equal to the first section of your finger, about an inch. Trimming is recommended every two to three months, or as needed.

8 Metamorphosis

Anyone who gazes at a healthy meadow can't help but be captivated by its beauty and fullness. The blades of grass are wide and strong, combining to form a wonderment of nature. But a pasture overcome with weeds and patches of unhealthy greenery is an eyesore.

Natural hair is analogous to a healthy, beautiful meadow. Hair that is free from chemicals can grow abundantly. Similar to a pasture overcome with weeds, chemically treated hair eventually will appear dry, limp, and patchy.

A metamorphosis can occur the first or second month after a relaxer has been applied to a child's scalp. If a parent decides to move a child to a natural hairstyle and away from dependence on relaxers, over time the point where new growth ends and the relaxed portions begin starts to tangle and break. The new growth will continue to rise and stand strong, while the relaxed hair will hang limp, tangled, and defeated.

This is the start of the metamorphosis.

In order to achieve a full head of naturally thick, beautiful hair, chemically treated hair must be removed. Only then can the hair flourish in its natural

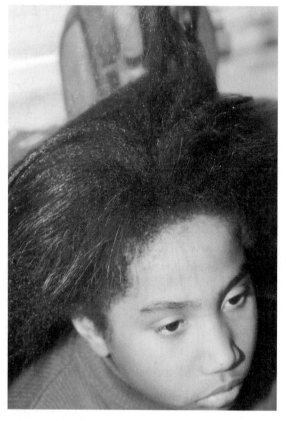
Chemically treated hair can appear limp and dry.

state. Otherwise the natural, healthy hair begins to split where the relaxed hair is breaking off.

I've styled and maintained the hair of many children whose parents are confused about what's happening to their child's hair during this transition. Often, parents think that they are doing the right thing by relaxing the hair again, thinking the hair will be more manageable and cause the child less pain. But with a little bit of patience and new knowledge, you and your child can embrace natural healthy hair.

Fortunately, many styling options are available during this transitional phase. Braided styles and styles that use synthetic and human hair extensions look good on transitioning hair. See Chapters 11 and 19.

Please understand: *There is no magic way to remove chemicals from your child's hair.* The safest and most effective method of removal is to cut off all of the relaxed hair. Immediate removal of relaxed hair will prevent split ends and further hair loss.

It's important to bolster your child's confidence during this time. Be prepared for the possibility that girls may be teased about their hair while it is short. Show your daughter pictures of beautiful women who have short hair, such as India Arie, Erykah Badu, and actress N'Bushe Wright. Compliment her on how short hair brings out her beautiful facial features. Think about getting special earrings that complement her hair, face, and head shape.

For those parents who are concerned about sacrificing their child's hair length, another option is to remove the relaxed hair gradually. Some parents prefer to cut off an inch a month until the chemically treated hair is all gone. If you choose to cut the chemicals in intervals, your child's hair can be cut at its rate of growth, so the hair you cut will not be missed.

Still, transitioning to natural hair gradually can be a frustrating experi-

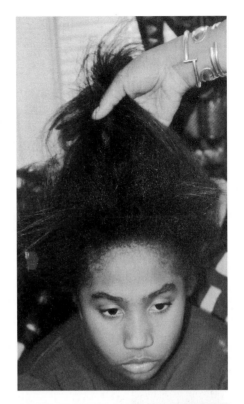

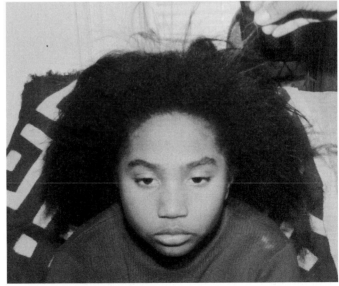

If a parent has already relaxed a child's hair and chooses not to relax the new growth, the point between the new growth and relaxed portions start to tangle and break.

43

ence for you and your child if you extend the metamorphosis before allowing the hair to achieve its natural state.

Also, keeping the relaxed hair as the natural hair grows in will cause the ends of the natural hair to start off damaged, which is why it's better to cut off all the relaxed hair at once. The compromise to save length results in some sacrifice to the health of your child's hair. Removing chemicals from the hair permanently will alleviate the sores, scabs, breakage, and burning of the scalp that are by-products of relaxing, texturizing, and excessive heat.

Transitional Denial

You and your child may experience "transitional denial" when you become frustrated during this period because you want results quickly. This can result in actions that will impede your progress toward a beautiful head of natural hair.

Transitional denial can take on various forms and extend the time it takes to transition to natural hair. Parents in this mindset sometimes turn to pressing and curling, believing that these actions aren't damaging. But they are. Straightening your child's hair with a hot comb can be extremely harmful. Instruments that are too hot can cause irreparable damage to hair and skin, and the hair will be unable to revert back to its kinky state. Again, the hair is left permanently straight and stringy.

Many parents believe that if they test the curling irons and hot combs on paper bags or paper towels and the paper doesn't turn brown, then the irons are safe to use on a child's hair. But they are wrong. Heat-damaged hair, like chemically damaged hair, will eventually have to be removed.

Another sign of transitional denial is making the decision to put texturizers in a child's hair. As children are going "natural," impatient parents feel that a texturizer will make their hair more manageable. Although texturizers curl the hair and relaxers straighten the hair, texturizers contain the same chemicals found in relaxers. Texturizers are ultimately damaging to the hair because they contain harsh chemicals that can cause hair loss and breakage. Ultimately, for a metamorphosis to occur, the texturized hair will have to to be cut off, just like the relaxed hair.

The curl pattern obtained by using a texturizer can be replicated by natural wet-set styles, such as two-strand twists, coils sets, and straw sets. This natural option is explained in Chapter 11.

Another form of transitional denial is the belief that something can be put into the hair to strip out the relaxer. Old wives tales include myths like using vinegar and lemon juice to remove a relaxer from hair. Relaxing the hair is a chemical process that actually changes the chemical bonds in the hair. *This change is permanent and irreversible.* The hair must be cut to safely remove the relaxer.

Ultimately, transitional denial further damages your child's hair and prolongs the metamorphosis process. Please be calm and patient. Working with natural-care products and abolishing heating implements and chemicals will lead to healthy, thick, natural hair. Locks, coils, braids, two-strand twists, and Afros are among the many wonderful natural hairstyles waiting for your child in a chemical-free future.

Perseverance will pay off if you keep the health of your child's hair in mind. My friend April gave her daughter, Amber, her first relaxer at the age of seven. Like many parents, April was ignorant about the natural beauty of kinky hair. She thought Amber's hair was nappy and hard to comb, so she chose to relax it. "I wanted my daughter's hair to be soft, smooth, and easy to comb," April recalled.

Three weeks after relaxing Amber's hair, April noticed hair breakage at the nape of Amber's neck. A week later, the breakage had spread all around the hairline.

"I wasn't in denial, and knew right away it was the relaxer," April said. She knew that she and Amber had to be patient and allow nature to take its course. Amber's hair needed to grow in naturally, free of all chemicals. April felt badly and wished she could undo the damage.

Amber's hair was in a bad state: Her hair was choppy and uneven; the hairline was thin and her hair was hard and brittle. April said she was embarrassed for her daughter and was harassed by friends and family members who wanted her to put another relaxer in Amber's hair. April said she tried to explain to people that the chemicals in the relaxers were the reason for Amber's hair damage. Fortunately for Amber, her mother held firm and refused to let ignorance prevail. Vowing never to put another relaxer in Amber's hair, April cut the relaxed hair off and taught herself how to braid. She braided Amber's hair back to health, styling it into two-strand twists and cornrows.

9 Quick and Easy Styles

This chapter is dedicated to all parents and caregivers who barely have enough time to get themselves ready for work in the morning, leaving little time to groom their children's hair. With practice, you can end frustration over morning hair grooming. Take some time out to familiarize yourself with these techniques. The more practice you have, the better you'll get.

Individual Basic Braiding

The phrase "individual braids" will be used here interchangeably with box braids, single braids, and plaits.

1. Begin with your hands close to the scalp, pulling tightly, but not too tightly. Separate the hair into three equal sections—one, two, and three, from left to right. It is very important that the sections are the same size. Cross section one (left) under section two. Section one is now in

the middle. Section two is now on the left. Cross section three (on the right) under the section in the middle (one). Place the hair on the left under the middle section. Now the middle is on the left and the left is the middle.

2. Take the section on the right and put it under the middle section, repeating this pattern to the end.

3. When you get near the end of the hair, you may find one of the hair sections is longer than the other sections. Simply borrow hair from the longer section, making all sections even, to complete the individual braid.

When you're first starting to braid, practice using larger sections of hair to make thicker braids. Before you realize it, you'll work more quickly and with more confidence and be better able to make smaller braids.

With practice, cornrows and individual braids are a cinch. Again, the key to good-looking braids is making sure you evenly distribute the hair into three equal parts.

Cornrows

Two Large Cornrows

Cornrows may appear to be a bit intimidating, but with practice, skilled perfection can follow within fifteen minutes to an hour. (The difference between cornrows and single braids are cornrows are attached to the scalp whereas individuals are single braids that freely move in different directions.)

1. Part the hair in the center of the scalp. Starting at the hairline, pick up three even sections of hair from the side that you're working with. The other side should be pinned and clipped.

2. Your palms should be facing your child's head. This is the key; you will be using several fingers as you figure out your own technique.

3. Securely hold all three strands of hair while crossing the sections of hair, using the same instructions for braiding. As you braid, moving down the head, pick up loose hair and add it into the braid, keeping the hair close to the scalp.

4. Unclip other side of hair and repeat steps 2 and 3.

Advanced Cornrows

Once you practice, you can advance with any braided hairstyle. Simply use smaller sections of hair. When creating smaller cornrows, keep the braids close together. Follow the instructions given for two large cornrows.

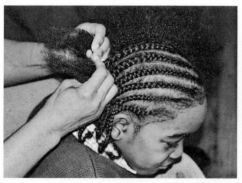

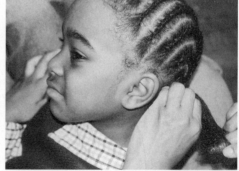

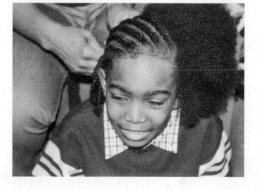

For thinner cornrows, simply use smaller sections of hair while following the general techniques for braiding. Securely hold all three strands of hair while crossing the sections of hair. Pick up loose hair and add it into the braid, keeping hair close to the scalp.

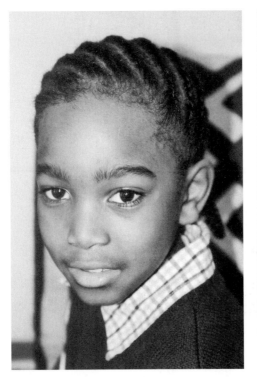

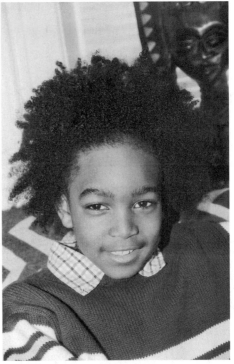

Amir sports cornrows.

After the cornrows have been taken out, Amir gives us a mini-Maxwell look with a major 'fro.

Twists

Two Strand-Twists

This is a quick and easy style that's truly simple. This style takes ten to twenty-five minutes depending on the size of the twists. This style is so versatile that we have four photos with styling options.

This hairstyle can be accomplished dry or wet and is great for swimming. Only keep this style in your child's hair for about two to three weeks.

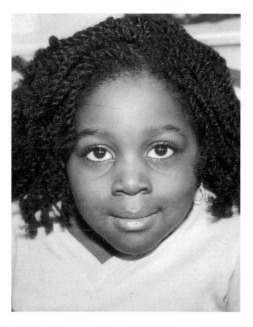 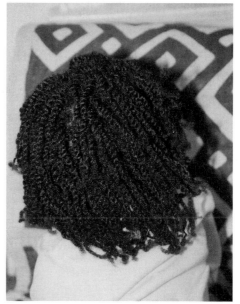

Two-strand twist-out in one ponytail.

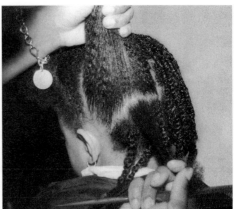

Step #2.

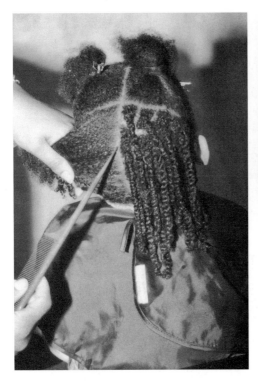

Step #1.

1. Once the hair is combed through, using your hair clips, separate a small section of hair, about the size of a quarter.

2. Then divide the hair into two even pieces.

3. Crisscross the right piece over the left piece and repeat this process until you get to the ends. The twist should resemble a rope.

4. If the hair is wet while you are styling it, it will naturally curl on the ends, sealing the twist. If you choose to blow dry your daughter's hair first, then you can secure the ends with a barrette if her hair doesn't stay together at the ends.

Practice makes perfect. Soon you will be able to make the twists smaller. With time, you will increase your speed.

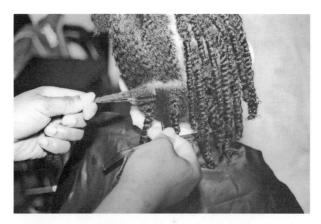

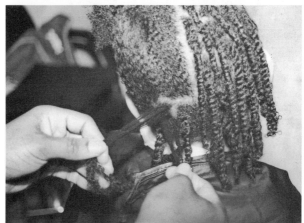

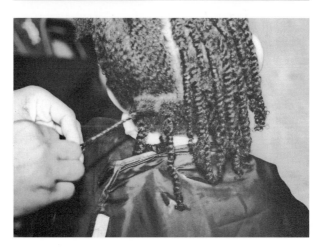

Step #3.

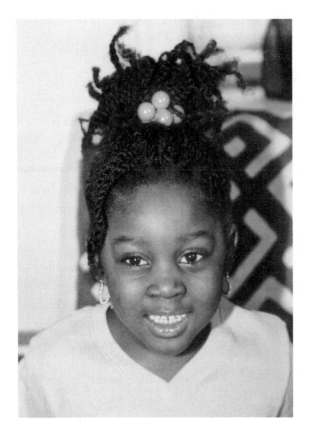

Two-strand twists in a ponytail.

Two-Strand Twist-Out

The two-strand twist-out is the two-strand twist neatly untwisted. (Try saying that five times fast.) This style is created by separating each twist at the root of the hair and splitting the twist apart. This is a fun style that adds a fuller look to your daughter's hair.

This style can't get wet, however. If it does, the hair will get puffy and start to swell and lose its shape. Below are three styling options for two-strand twists. This only takes a few minutes.

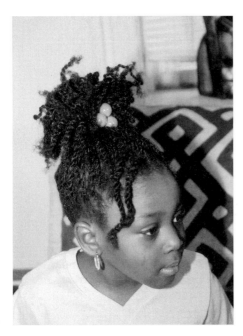

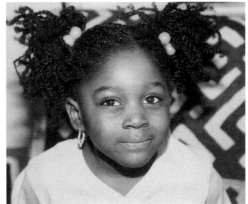

Two-strand twists in two ponytails.

Two-strand twists in one ponytail.

* TWIST-OUT 'FRO—carefully untwist the two-strand twists to create one ponytail puff.
* ONE PONYTAIL—gently pull up twists and place a ballie (an elastic band with a colorful ball on each end) or other hair ornament around it.
* TWO PONYTAILS—gather two sections together and place a ballie or hair ornament around it.

Ponytail Two-Twist Buns

1. Part the hair into two sections. Using your boar-bristle brush, brush the hair into a neat ponytail.
2. Put the ballie around the section of hair, close to the scalp.
3. Separate the hair into two sections and twist the hair into a larger two-strand twist.
4. Twist the hair all the way to the end.
5. Wrap the end of the twist around the ballie, until the hair bun is secure. (Use hair pins to hold the hair if the hair is too short.)
6. Follow steps 3 to 5 on the other side of the head.

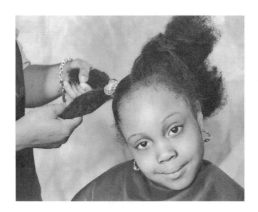

Step #3.

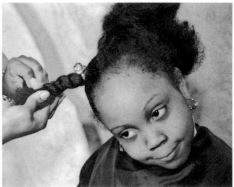

Step #4.

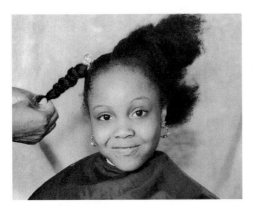

Step #4 *(continued).*

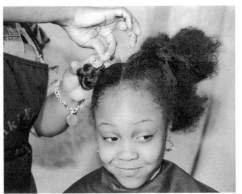

Step #5.

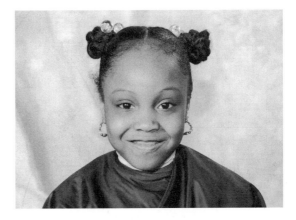

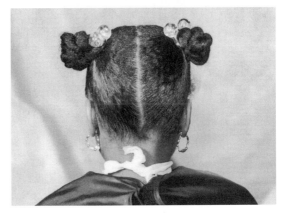

Finished ponytail two-twist buns.

57

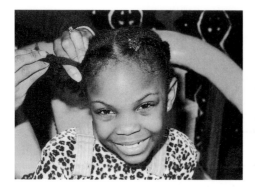
Step #3.

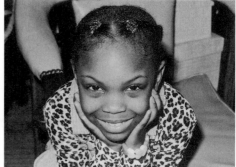
Finished flat twists.

Flat Twists

This style is similar to cornrowing. Instead of using three sections of hair, you start off with two sections.

1. Make a center part in your child's hair.
2. Clip one side of the hair out of the way.
3. Starting at the hairline, grab two sections.
4. Using two pieces of hair, crisscross the right section over the left section.
5. Pick up hair and add it into each section you crisscross, keeping the hair close to the scalp as in a cornrow.
6. When you reach the end of the section you're working with, continue twisting the hair down. (This might become a free-floating braid.) When you reach the end, secure the hair with a barrette.

Afro Puffs

Afro puffs are fun and easy. Remember the key to this style is making sure the hair is thoroughly combed through.

1. Brush the hair to the center of your daughter's head.
2. Securely wind a ballie around her hair twice.
3. Using your wide-tooth comb, pick out the Afro.

You can also vary the style a bit by braiding your daughter's bangs and creating a ponytail puff with the remainder of hair.

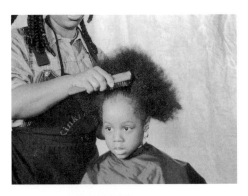
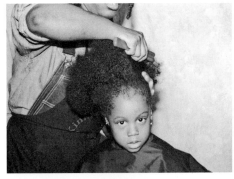
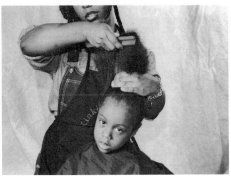
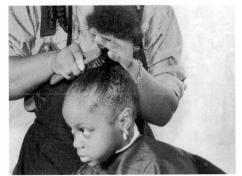

Step #1.

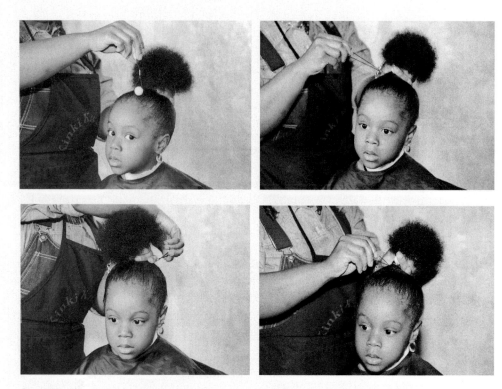

Step #2.

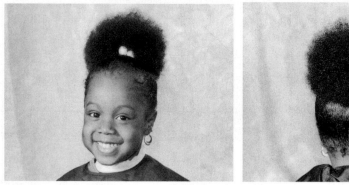

Finished afro puff.

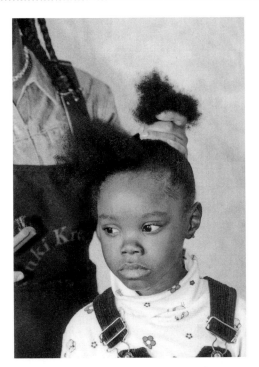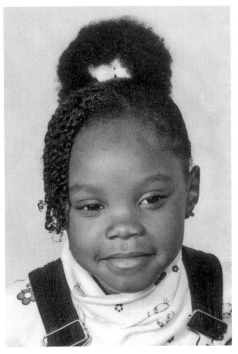

You can braid your daughter's bangs to wear with her pontytail puff.

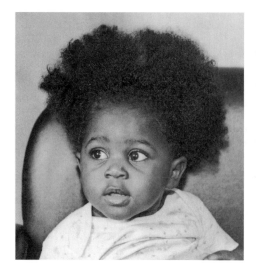

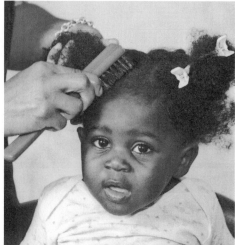

Step #1.

Two Ponytail Puffs

1. Part the hair into two sections.
2. Repeat afro-puff steps 2 and 3 for each section, this time using a center part.

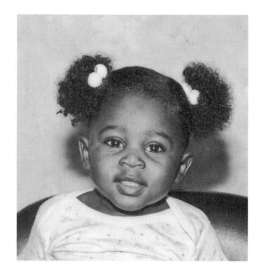

Finished ponytail puffs.

10 Beading and Ornaments

It's a common African-American cultural practice to adorn hair with various beads, barrettes, cowrie shells, and ribbons. These adornments add beauty and completion to a hairstyle.

Here are step-by-step instructions on stringing beads onto braids and properly putting ornaments on the hair.

Materials needed:

* Thin Wire
* String
* Beads, barrettes, cowrie shells, and/or ribbons

While braids can be squeezed through a large-enough bead (this is old school and time consuming), stringing on beads is a quicker process.

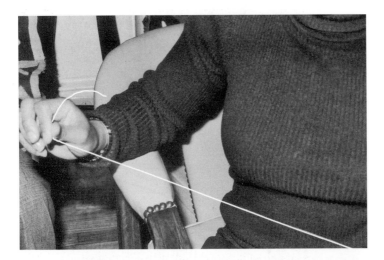

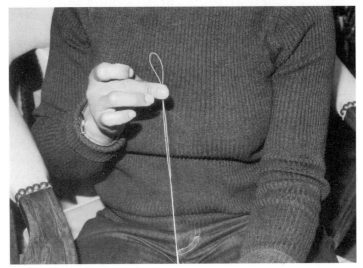

Step #1.

1. Get a firm piece of string, about 12 inches long, and a bead. Fold the string in half.
2. Join the open ends of the string together. Thread them through the hole of a bead and tie a secure knot. This bead will stop all the other beads from sliding off the string.

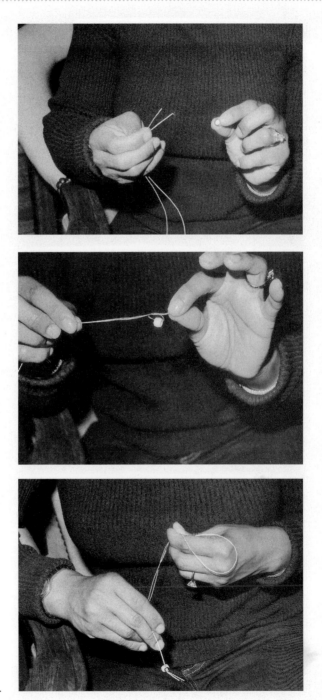

Step #2.

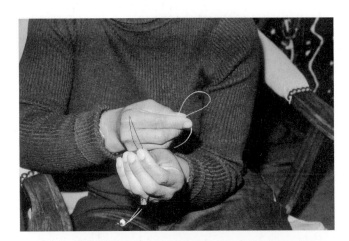

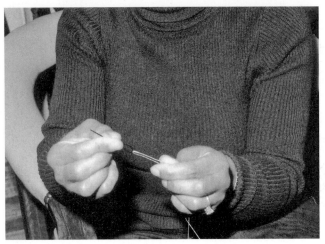

Step #3.

3. Fold a piece of wire in half and hook it at the loop end of the string so that the wire is extended.
4. String the beads through the wire and let them drop to the bottom bead. Continue this process until the desired amount of beads have been used, leaving at least two inches at the top of the loop.

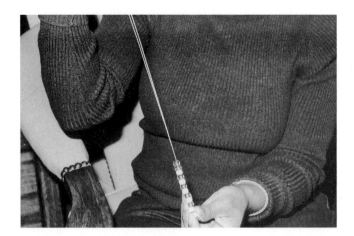

Step #4.

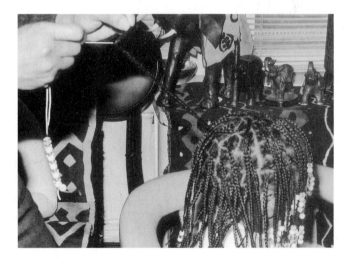

Step #6.

5. Remove the wire, while holding the string securely.

6. Take the end of a braid and place it through the loop (be sure that the hole of the bead is large enough to fit over the braid).

7. Fold the braid in half. Staying close to the end of the braid while holding the braid firmly, push the desired amount of beads onto the braid.

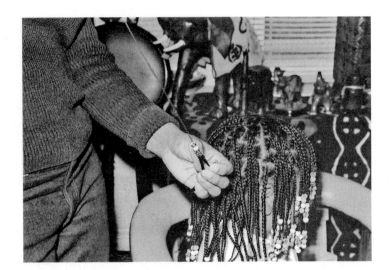

Step #7.

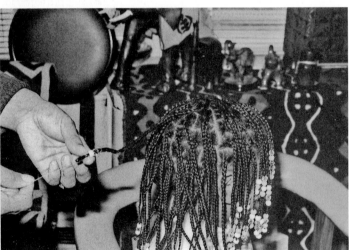

Step #8.

8. Remove the string from the beads. Be careful not to drop them.

9. Pull one bead down close to the end of the braid.

10. Take a piece of wire, about three to four inches long, and stick it through the bottom bead. Leaving a half inch of wire visible, fold the wire over

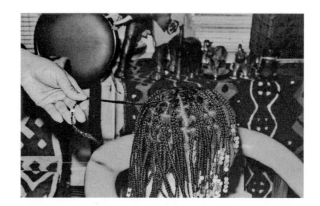

Step #9.

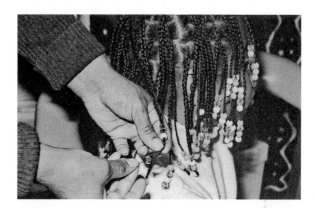

Step #10.

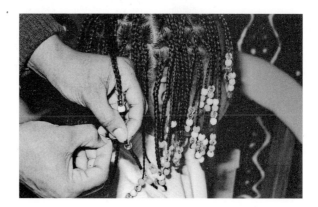

Step #11.

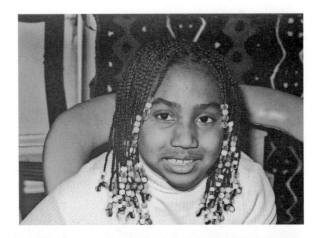

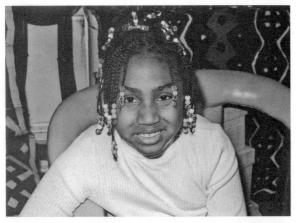

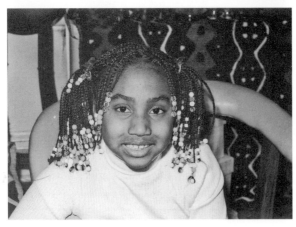

Finished beautifully
beaded hair.

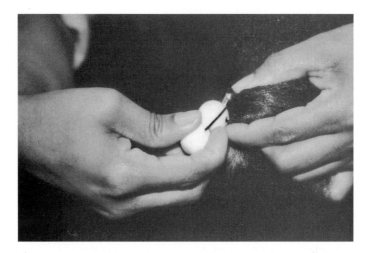

When using ballies as hair ornaments, hold the hair firmly in your hand. Using the other hand, hold one ball and wrap it twice around the hair. Fasten the ballie by stretching the first ball over the second ball.

the bead, holding the wire firmly. Wrap the wire around the top of the braid.

11. Pull the rest of the beads down, covering the wire.

If beading's not for you, there are a variety of hair ornaments that can be used to make any hairstyle complete. Ornaments are like icing on a cake. Ornaments that have elasticity are usually the best choices. If you choose to use barrettes, make sure that they don't have any metal on them. Metal can pull out the hair over a period of time.

If the braid or ponytail is too thick, then you run the risk of the barrette popping off. Wrap the end of the braid around the inside of the barrette three or four times. This will secure the barrette.

71

11 Daily Maintenance

Daily maintenance is important in the upkeep of all hairstyles. Depending on the style, upkeep can preserve the style two to four weeks.

Wrap a silk or satin scarf over your child's hair at night to hold the hair neatly in place. Wearing the scarf will also help protect your child's hair from breaking off. Be careful not to use a cotton scarf or one made from Lycra, because these fabrics tend to pull hair out.

Also stay away from sponge hair-rollers. Your child's hair can get caught in the sponge, causing hair breakage.

For a curlier look, you can always try a braid set. Using your spray bottle, wet the hair with water and braid the hair into large sections. Allow the hair to dry four to seven hours. Unbraid, and the hair will be curly.

It's also important to oil your child's scalp every three or four days, or as needed. If your child's hair starts to get dry sooner, than add oil earlier. To avoid clogging pores, don't oversaturate the scalp with oil. Too much oil can also slow down hair's growth process. A teaspoonful of oil should be sufficient. Use a little more if the child has a large scalp.

If the hair along your child's hairline starts to curl up and you want to go for a neater look, simply apply a small amount of hair gel (use a clear all-natural gel that doesn't contain any alcohol) at the hairline and brush the hair back. Then, tie a scarf around the head, covering the hairline as well, and let the gel sit overnight.

12 Braid Removal and Shampooing Braids

Removing Braids

Depending on the size of the braid, you will be using a rattail comb or your fingers to remove the braids. If the braids are thin, use a rattail comb; if the braids are thick, use your fingers. If your daughter or son has had their hair braided by a professional at a hair salon, keep in mind most salons provide braid removal for varying prices.

If you choose to remove the braids yourself, here are a few tips.

1. For extensions, cut the extension braid near where your child's natural hair ends. So that you don't cut your child's natural hair, estimate about three inches longer than your child's natural hair and cut the extension there.

2. Using the tail end of your rattail comb, repeatedly pierce the center of the braid, separating the hair until you reach the top. There may be hard

crust and debris where the natural hair and extension meet. Don't comb this part. Combing could rip the hair out of its follicle and cause serious damage to your child's hair and scalp. Simply gently separate the debris and hair strands with your fingers. If there is too much crust, lightly spray the area using your oil and water solution to soften the area and make it easier to manage. Do not oversaturate the hair; oversaturation can cause the hair to tangle.

3. After you have removed a cluster of braids, comb through that section of hair, then twist or braid the section and clip the section out of the way.

4. Repeat this technique until the braids are completely removed.

Removing braids requires skill and patience. Rushing through this process will cause you to rip your child's hair out, resulting in pain and unnecessary hair loss.

Shampooing braids

For more elaborate braided styles that were completed by a professional stylist, I recommend consulting that stylist about the best procedures to use for shampooing that style. For simpler braided styles, use a shampoo that is clear and doesn't contain any conditioner.

1. Mix eight ounces of warm water with one ounce of shampoo. This solution is best for braids because the shampoo will be equally distributed through the braids with no globs.

2. Shampoo the hair, gently massaging the scalp. Do not use a conditioner, since it's difficult to completely remove conditioner from braids. Conditioners tend to cake up in the hair and then attract dirt and debris.

3. Rinse the hair thoroughly. You'll know when you're done rinsing because the water should be clear.

4. Repeat steps 2 and 3.
5. Towel dry and/or use a blow-dryer to help remove some of the dampness.
6. Finally, wrap your child's hair with a silk or satin scarf to smooth down the frizzies (stray hairs that stand out from the braid).
7. Add a small amount of oil to the scalp to replenish the oil lost in washing. Then massage a tablespoonful of oil onto the braids for a nice sheen.

Note: Don't try to brush braids. This can cause breakage.

Dry Shampoo

We suggest a dry shampoo for any style you are keeping in more than two weeks. Some braided styles can last two to eight weeks.

1. Apply witch hazel or Sea Breeze astringent to a cotton ball and rub the cotton ball in between the sectioned parts of the scalp.
2. Allow to dry and then apply oil to the scalp.

13 Boys

There has been a long-standing tradition in the African-American community that it's taboo to cut your son's hair before he's one year old. Some parents wait even longer, choosing not to cut a male child's hair until he's old enough to ask for a different style. The tradition is a good one; you shouldn't cut a child's hair until the child is at least one or two years of age.

Before one or two, the child's hair is still maturing, developing into its natural texture and form. If you cut your son's hair too early, it could damage growth. The sharp edge of the clippers used to cut hair, when used close to the scalp lines of undeveloped hair, can permanently alter your child's natural hairline.

At age one, the hair is strong enough for a child to receive a first haircut. But cutting the hair this early is optional. Many parents choose to allow their sons' hair to grow until the age of five or later. There is no definitive rule on when you must cut your son's hair. If you choose to keep his hair long, you can braid or twist it. Boys nowadays have a variety of styles they can wear.

Although boys don't need the same amount of attention when it comes to

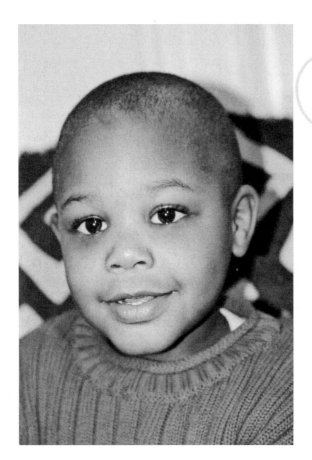

hair care as girls do, since many wear their hair short, boys' hair shouldn't go unattended. For boys and girls, the same maintenance routine is recommended. (See Chapter 11.)

It is strongly recommended that you send your son to a professional barbershop that caters to young children, where the barber will be patient and understanding if your son is uncomfortable and afraid, for his first haircut. If possible, take your son to the shop prior to his appointment and let him become familiar with the shop, the chair, the barber, and the equipment.

Try to make sure your consultation is on a not-so-busy day. Ask your barber if your son can hold the clippers and examine them because clippers make

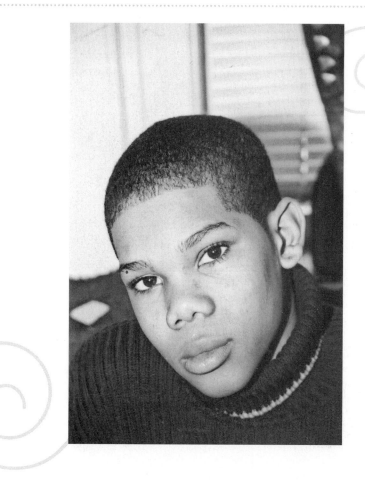

noise, which can scare a child. Holding the clippers will help most boys feel relaxed.

Here are some tips to make the barbershop experience a good one:

* Some barbers offer shampoo services at the barbershop, but sometimes shampooing can be a lot to ask of a busy barber.
* If shampoos are not offered, then a sure way to help your barber is to shampoo your child's hair before he goes to the barbershop.
* Combing your son's hair through thoroughly before the visit will ensure a less painful haircut.

* Getting your son's hair cut for the first time can be an extremely emotional experience. Your son will lose his babyish look and start to look like a little man. When introducing the child to his first haircut, it's important not to show negative emotions. And it's important when you see your son looking like a little man not to overreact.

* Concentrate on showing encouraging support. If you are calm, then your son will be calm.

* Take before-and-after pictures and ask your barber for a lock of your child's hair to save as a memento.

* Be prepared to assist your barber in the haircut. If the barber needs you to help control your child while performing the haircut, then the barber will tell you so. Otherwise, let your barber make all of the calls.

* Don't be alarmed if the barber holds your child's head firmly while performing the haircut. Sometimes this is necessary when handling small children, and it doesn't hurt. Holding a child firmly is often necessary in order to help the barber give a good haircut with even lines.

* A barber shouldn't give the child an outline with clippers until the child is three to five years old. Outlines can cause permanent sores, scabs, and scratches, and may interfere with the natural development of the child's hairline.

* Never allow a razor outline until the child is at least twelve or thirteen. A razor is too sharp and, after a period of time, the razor could leave a permanent mark on the forehead. Barber clippers can achieve the same look.

* Licensed barbers are professional and experienced. They know what they are doing, so allow them to exhibit their skills and practice their craft.

* After your child has received his haircut, remove all of the loose hairs by brushing them out and shampoo the hair.

* Massage a teaspoonful of oil all over the child's hair and use a soft bristle-brush to brush the hair back in place.

* It's always important to take your time when combing your son's hair. Don't rake rapidly or roughly through the child's hair.

* If you are having a difficult time getting the comb through his hair, use a wider tooth comb or spray a little water on the hair to help the comb move along. Boys and girls should never feel pain when they are having their hair groomed.
* Oil the hair and scalp every three to four days, but be sure not to over-saturate.
* Always practice good sanitation at home. Make sure your son has his own comb and brush. Clean his comb and brush with shampoo and water every time you shampoo his hair.

Boys have plenty of choices when it comes to styles. Haircuts are an option, but some boys want longer hair. My son Andre refers to braids that have length as "hang time." There are a couple of hairstyles for boys that you can choose from in Chapter 20.

14 Locks and Maintenance

Locks are naturally textured strands of hair intertwined and meshed together into tubular shapes of various sizes. Locks are often thought of as a low-maintenance style—that's true after your hair is already locked, but it can take three months to a year to lock your hair depending on hair texture. It is a process that can be difficult to maintain (especially at the beginning) because it takes time, skill, and patience. If you choose to lock your child's hair yourself, I strongly recommend you take classes on locking from a salon that specializes in natural hair care. If you take classes, you can learn how to properly trim and shampoo your child's locks.

Keep in mind that shampooing your child's locks every two to three weeks is extremely important because dirt and debris can get trapped inside the intertwined hair in a lock. If this continues to happen and the debris builds up, the lock could become dusty and start to smell sour. Locks that are tended to regularly will offer your child a sculpted, manicured, and stylized look.

In between visits at the hair salon, you may want to groom your child's locks. Before starting, you'll need:

* A large scrunchie
* Spray bottle containing six parts water and one part oil
* Hair clips
* Oil
* Natural hair gel
* Shears

1. Lightly oil the scalp and hair. Massage the oil thoroughly into the scalp and hair.
2. Start from the nape of the neck. Use the large scrunchie or clips to hold the locks you are not working with out of the way.
3. Mist the section you are working with, using your water and oil solution.
4. Working with one lock at a time, apply a small amount of gel at the root of the lock and drag the gel down to the end of the lock.
5. Sometimes, the locks web or tangle together at the roots. Don't pull the locks apart. Use your shears to cut any strings of hair, which will allow the lock to separate into its own section.
6. Roll the lock between your palms until the lock seems to be tight at the root. (Be careful not to twist too tightly, since this could cause breakage.)
7. Clip the lock down and repeat these steps for the rest of the locks.

Here are a few additional tips:

* If your child's scalp becomes dirty, you can give your child a dry shampoo using witch hazel on a cotton ball to cleanse the scalp. Remember to add a small amount of oil to the scalp.
* You can have variety even with locks. Here's a style to try: Saturate your child's hair with your oil and water solution and take large sections of the locks and braid them together. Leave the large braids in overnight and

unbraid them in the morning. You now have a beautifully crinkled set of locks.

* Remember that locks cannot be combed through. We shed approximately one hundred strands of hair per day. Because you do not comb or brush locks, none of the shedding hair is combed or brushed out so the shedding hair starts to wind around the lock like a vine. This is why locks grow so long.

15 Choosing the Right Salon

One of the best ways to find the salon that is right for you and your child is word of mouth. Ask around. In your travels throughout the day, while you're in the grocery store, bookstore, or anyplace children may be accompanying their parents, pay close attention to other children's hairstyles. Inquire about a style you like. Sometimes, a parent will have a stylist's card with them and they'll usually be happy to share information about where they've had a good experience.

You want to find a salon that has a great reputation for working with children. Find out how long they have been in business. A year is long enough for a reputation to be established and for you to feel secure. When looking for the right salon, be sure to call around and ask if they take children and about the starting age. There are some salons that do good work, but they may not be child friendly. This could cause the stylist, you, and your child to be uncomfortable. So plan ahead. Remind yourself that you have a little child who wants a perfect hairstyle, and you want a healthy, natural hairstyle for her.

Consultation

Ask the salon if they offer consultations. This gives the stylist the opportunity to check the texture and condition of your child's hair and discuss style options with you. Most salons have books you can look through that are filled with a variety of styles to choose from.

The consultation should also include information about the price of the style, an explanation of the technique, and an estimated length of time it will take for the style to be completed, including any waiting time. Also ask about how long the style will last and its maintenance requirements.

During the consultation, you shouldn't feel rushed. A stylist can answer questions even while working on someone else's hair. Don't feel intimidated. Ask all of the questions you came with and continue the dialogue until you feel satisfied.

Engaging a stylist who agrees to a consultation is important because it suggests that the stylist cares enough to learn about your child. It also provides you with an opportunity to check out the salon environment and see if it's a place you'd feel comfortable bringing your child and perhaps leaving him or her for a while.

Taking your child to a hair salon for the first time can be a fun experience and can also be considered an important rite of passage. Usually, children are pretty excited about going to a salon for the first time—until they actually get in the chair. Sometimes, the excitement turns into fear once the child is separated from the parent and is experiencing a stranger touching them. The child can feel a sense of abandonment if the parent doesn't stay nearby on that first salon visit, so it's a good idea to stay close.

Here are a few tips to help prepare the child for the new experience:

* Have a talk with your child a few weeks before and start continuously preparing her for the salon experience. Assure your daughter that it's important for her to be a big girl who can cooperate and collaborate with a

hair professional and, in return, her hair will be styled beautifully by a stylist who has the skills to make her hair look magnificent.

* It can be tough watching your daughter getting braids, or your son receive his first haircut, but it's important for you to cooperate with the stylist as well. Assist the stylist (if asked) without too much interference. That's why you had the consultation, so that you and the stylist would be clear about the services agreed upon and so that you would feel comfortable.

* Before you and your child leave, be sure to ask the stylist to tell you how to maintain the new hairstyle. Also find out what hair products your stylist recommends and if there are any brand preferences.

* If your child starts to cry or scream, ask the stylist if you can hold your child's hand or let the child sit on your lap. A parent came into Kiddie Kreations with her four-year-old daughter. The woman said her daughter had been excited about having her hair braided. I asked the little girl whether she was excited and she replied, "Yes."

I sat the little girl in my chair, draped her in a cape, and began to comb her hair. The little girl started crying hysterically. I asked her what was wrong and she screamed louder. Her mother instructed me to continue combing her hair despite her daughter's screams and tears.

While wiping her daughter's tears, the mother said "Didn't you beg to have your hair done? You said you were going to be a good girl. Do you want to leave?"

Ignoring every word, the little girl reached for her mother to pick her up. I suggested that the mother sit in the chair and hold her daughter on her lap. I was able to successfully finish the child's hair. This approach worked twice, and by her third visit, the little girl sat in my chair by herself. This is one of the many inspirations for the existence of Kiddie Kreations. Children sometimes have special needs that require time and patience.

16 Teenagers

Once your daughter becomes a teenager, she usually goes through a rite of passage with her hair while undergoing social, physical, and emotional changes.

Hairstyling may become a major factor in her life as she develops increased concern about her appearance. At the same time, this is when peer pressure kicks in. She is trying to get in touch with who she is while also having to deal with what others think. For parents who have chosen natural hairstyles for their daughters, life with your teenage daughter will likely become a challenge. She will want to change her youthful hairstyle to a more mature hairstyle, and she may also feel pressured to change from a natural style.

When teenagers go through puberty, they start to stray away from their mom and dad's ideas of aesthetics. Young people's sense of style and beauty changes. In the case of my friend April and her daughter, Amber, April allowed her daughter to eat the entire pig before she realized it was pork.

Six years after April had stopped using relaxers and started braiding Amber's hair, Amber became a teenager, and her mother faced another hair challenge. At age thirteen, Amber came home from school one day and asked

April if she could get her hair relaxed. April told her no, and explained that relaxers were too harsh and they cause breakage and hair damage.

Amber began to protest, saying she didn't want to wear her hair in braids or other natural hairstyles anymore. Amber wanted to look more mature, and she associated straight hair with maturity. Amber reminded her mother that all of her friends had relaxed hair and asked why couldn't she. April responded, "When you turn eighteen years old, then you have permission to destroy your hair, and that's final."

Under duress, Amber continued wearing braids and natural hairstyles that were slightly altered (no more barrettes and ribbons) to fit her age. This kept Amber satisfied for the moment.

But Amber constantly pleaded for a straighter look that was more like the styles the other teenaged girls were wearing. Finally, April and Amber came up with a compromise: Amber could straighten her hair with a hot-iron comb.

Still, the excessive heat from the hot-iron comb started causing severe breakage to Amber's hair. April knew this would happen, but it was important for Amber to see it for herself. Amber, older now, was able to experience what her mother had tried to protect her from. She was of course upset that her hair started breaking and soon developed a new appreciation for natural, healthy hair. Amber has finally embraced natural hair and loves to style her hair in braids and cornrows.

April is a professional natural stylist at Kinki Kreations Braiding Salon and Amber, who is learning to braid, sometimes answers the phones and schedules appointments.

This story reflects how difficult it can be for parents and teenagers to withstand the weight of peer pressure. As parents, we have a responsibility to guide our children to make the right decisions. It took patience and tolerance to get Amber to see what her mother already knew. But sometimes children have to experience something to really learn it.

17 Dandruff and Scalp Disorders

Dandruff can be the result of many factors. It comes from poor circulation, poor nutrition, poor hydration, and stress and tension. It also is caused by not cleansing the scalp properly, infrequent shampooing, and the use of heavy grease, creams, and gels on the hair and scalp.

The medical term for dandruff is pityriasis. It is recognizable by large flakes clearly visible on the scalp. Dandruff usually itches. Although daily shampooing may provide some relief, it can be counterproductive. Daily shampooing is stressful on the hair and extremely drying, causing the hair to become brittle and break.

Dandruff can be a very severe health problem. If you are experiencing uncontrollable dandruff, if your scalp is bleeding, or if there is pus coming from the scalp, you should consult a physician.

There are two types of severe dandruff that require medical attention:

* PITYRIASIS STEATOIDES (oily dandruff)—Greasy, waxy, large yellowish scales combined with sebum (pus-like oil) that causes the dandruff to

stick to the hair and scalp. When this type of dandruff is lifted and removed with a comb, bleeding or pus occurs in the infected and inflamed area.

 * PITYRIASIS CAPITIS SIMPLEX (dry dandruff)—This dandruff is highly contagious and looks like large white flakes. It's important to talk to your children about not sharing hats, combs, brushes, hair ornaments, or any other article used on the head or scalp. Get into the habit of cleaning all hair tools with a 70 percent alcohol solution for ten to fifteen minutes. This will sanitize all implements.

If these conditions exist, seek medical attention from a dermatologist to diagnose the problem and get proper medication.

Treating a Child's Dandruff at Home

If the dandruff is not serious, you can consider taking care of it yourself. Using a cotton swab, ball, or fingers, you can massage tea tree oil, witch hazel, or Sea Breeze. But if your child's dandruff can't be cured by using these remedies, consult a physican before using dandruff shampoos.

When shampooing hair for dandruff control, look for shampoos that include sulfur as an active ingredient. Some of the shampoos that I have successfully used on my clients are Organic Root Stimulator, Praises Oil, and Sulfur 8. These shampoos should be diluted with water before applying them to your child's scalp: mix a quarter-size dollop of shampoo with a cup of water.

1. Carefully brush or comb up the flakes. This will help stimulate the scalp and get the blood flowing. If blood or pus is present, don't irritate the area. Allow the scalp to heal for up to two hours before cleansing the scalp with a dandruff shampoo; otherwise the shampoo could irritate the scalp and sting.

2. Shampoo the hair with medicated shampoo; gently massage the scalp

with the balls of your fingertips, making sure not to scratch. Medicated dandruff shampoos are strong. If excessive scratching has irritated the surface of the scalp, the shampoo could burn and sting the scalp, leaving the child in discomfort, even pain.

3. Leave the shampoo on the hair for five to fifteen minutes.
4. Rinse thoroughly with warm water.
5. Repeat steps 2 to 4.
6. Apply conditioner and allow the conditioner to stay on the hair for five to ten minutes.
7. Repeat step 4.
8. Towel dry the hair and add oil, then follow the steps for hair preparation in Chapter 7.

18 Just Ask Jena

Parents have many questions and concerns about their children's hair. Here are some common inquiries I've received. Hopefully you'll find your answers here.

1. **What is natural hair?**

   Natural hair is virgin hair that has not been chemically altered in texture and color.

2. **I straighten my daughter's hair with a straightening comb, but I haven't put any chemicals in her hair. Is my daughter's hair still considered natural?**

   Yes, your daughter's hair can indeed still be considered natural, but there are other issues. Often when children have their hair straightened with a hot comb, the comb is too hot. The hair becomes singed and breaks off. Any process using heat can damage the hair and cause a change in the hair's chemical composition.

3. What is the lifespan of hair?

The exact lifespan of hair is unknown, but it seems the average is two to seven years.

4. My child came home from school crying. She said that the other children teased her because she didn't have a relaxer. *Help!*

First explain to your child that natural hair is wonderful and heaven-sent. Educate your child about the negative effects of relaxers on the hair and about how relaxers can burn the scalp. Also show your child pictures of beautiful braided and natural hair styles on everyday people as well as recognized celebrities. If your child is old enough to understand, explain the historic downgrading of people of African descent and what that has meant in terms of appreciating the way we look and our hair's natural properties.

5. What are the best shampoos and conditioners for my child's hair?

The best shampoos and conditioners are the ones that are pH-balanced. They should have a moisturizer base and contain a detangler. Always read the ingredients. Your shampoo and conditioner should contain mostly water, herbs, and minerals.

6. My child's hair is extremely dry and brittle. What can I do?

First, is the hair really hard and brittle or is it healthy and strong? Don't expect natural hair to look or feel like relaxed hair. Natural hair has firm texture and strength. Dry hair is usually the result of improper diet, a lack of water, certain medications, and the use of harsh chemicals found in relaxers, perms, and hair color. So first and foremost, make sure your child is eating correctly and drinking enough water. Water helps to lubricate all parts of the body, including the hair.

To help alleviate dryness, use a deep conditioner following shampooing. Deep conditioners, the kind that you leave on for a few moments and wash out, will penetrate and protect the hair shaft while providing added moisture. Avoid leave-in conditioners because they tend to attract debris, leaving the hair dull and dusty-looking.

7.   My son is interested in having a texturizer put in his hair. Is it safe?

A texturizer is a milder form of a relaxer. It is just as damaging as a perm because it can cause the same damage—hair loss, baldness, and scalp sores. If your son wants a curlier, natural look to his hair, try a coil set, where you coil the hair with a rattail comb and pick it out with your fingers.

8.   My son wants to get his hair cornrowed, but it doesn't seem long enough. What can we do?

A great transitional hairstyle for young men while their hair grows is coils, which is what Deione, the boy model on this book's cover, is sporting. Another popular transitional hairstyle, popular with boys and girls, is braids achieved by adding synthetic extensions with the invisible stitch technique. (A professional should do this.)

You need to have at least three inches of hair to braid in order to create cornrows. Hair texture is also very important. Tightly textured hair only requires three inches of growth; hair that has a looser curl can require up to six inches of growth before cornrows can be achieved and maintained.

9.   My child has long, thick natural hair, and we both dread having to comb it. What can we do to make combing easier?

It is best to work with natural hair while it's wet. You'll need a wide-tooth comb and a spray bottle filled with six parts water and one part oil.

Spray the hair until it is saturated, then part it into four to eight sections. Clip off each section to keep it separated. Comb through each section individually, spraying again as needed. Remember to hold the hair firmly and comb the hair starting at the ends, working your way back up to the roots. It's important to twist or braid each section after you've combed it through so that the hair doesn't tangle while you work on other sections. Once this comb through is done, then you'll be able to style the hair using the natural styles. A detailed description of the comb-through process is offered in Chapter 7.

10. **My child's hairline is receding. What causes this?**

    A receding hairline is caused by overprocessing with chemicals and also by other kinds of physical stress on the hair. Pulling hair back into tight ponytails and too-tightly braided cornrows can cause traction alopecia, meaning you are literally pulling out the hair. Harsh chemicals, used to relax the hair, can break off the hair and burn the scalp, rendering the area permanently bald.

11. **What purpose do extensions serve?**

    Extensions serve several purposes. A braided or twisted style lasts twice as long when extensions are used because the synthetic or human hair material used keeps your child's hair sandwiched in between. The extended hair is stronger and able to keep its shape longer. Extensions protect your natural hair from breakage, and they add more fullness and versatility to a style. Extensions also can be used to help some people move through the transition period, making it possible to move from relaxed to natural hair without sacrificing length.

12. **What is the difference between human hair and synthetic hair extensions?**

    Human hair is versatile to style and can be set on rod rollers. It's also very light on the head and can be curled into different styles. Styling agents such as mousse and gel can be used on human hair. However, human hair does have drawbacks. It swells when it's washed, which may cause slippage at the point where the extensions are attached and make your style look like the extensions have been in longer than they have.

    Synthetic hair is an excellent choice for extensions. Synthetic hair is manmade and has superb longevity. Its styling versatility when plaited into individual braids is virtually endless. The use of styling agents is not recommended with synthetic hair because these agents can cause a flaky buildup and attract debris. However, synthetic hair can be washed successfully with no significant slippage.

A style using synthetic hair extensions lasts twice as long as a style using natural hair.

13. I would like for my child to wear braids with extensions. What is a safe and appropriate age to begin wearing this style?

    Extensions are safe any time after age three to five. Unless you have had practice in applying extensions before, it would be best to have a professional apply the extensions. Also, make sure you choose a style that is not too heavy. If you're not careful, too much hair can be too heavy on the child's head, causing neck problems and a potential receding hairline. Keep your child looking youthful. Some style suggestions are featured in Chapter 9.

14. What kind of comb do you recommend I use on my child's hair?

    A wide-tooth comb is usually an excellent choice. The tighter the hair texture, the wider the comb's teeth should be. This prevents hair from breaking during combing.

15. What is the difference between relaxers and perms?

    Relaxers actually "relax" the hair by making it straight instead of curly. Perms use a different chemical and make straight hair curly. Many people use the two words interchangeably, but African Americans actually relax their hair even though they may use the term perm *to describe the process.*

16. Is there a difference between an adult relaxer and a child's relaxer or perm?

    First off, a relaxer is just another name for a perm. The basic difference is that a child's perm is traditionally not as harsh as perms made for adults. However, both adult and child perms destroy the hair. Both are equally damaging to the hair and both can burn the scalp.

17. How long does it take for a relaxer to grow out?

    A relaxer never actually grows out of the hair, but the relaxed hair, which is really destroyed, eventually splits and breaks off. The best thing to do is to ei-

ther cut an inch of the hair once a month or just cut it all off and go all natural. Chapter 8 describes in detail how to make a successful and comfortable transition from relaxed to natural hair.

18. **My child's hair is broken off and damaged from relaxers. Help!**

Provided there is enough new growth, the best choice is to cut the relaxed hair off and proceed with a short natural hairstyle. You might consider how a short, attractive natural style shows off your child's face. A cute short 'fro, two-strand twists, cornrows, or braided or twisted styles that use extensions are among your options during this transitional period and later.

19. **Is hair grease good for natural hairstyles?**

The best thing for natural hair is to use a natural oil that contains herbs, olive oil, and other natural ingredients. Natural oils penetrate the hair and scalp and do not sit on top of the hair like heavy grease products, which tend to collect debris. Hair grease may also block hair follicles in the scalp if applied too heavily. The closed follicles will slow down the hair's growth process.

20. **What is the best oil for my child's hair?**

It's best to use oils that contain natural ingredients. We recommend products that contain some of the following ingredients: aloe, sage oil, olive oil, almond, lavender, rosemary, and castor oils, just to name a few. These products can be found at a natural hair salon or at a health food store.

21. **Is it normal for a child to cry as soon as he or she sees a comb or brush?**

Your child probably associates hair grooming with pain. Maybe your child has tender, injured scalp spots from old perms or maybe the child's hair has been pulled too tightly. It's always good to offer some positive words of reassurance. We suggest you use a wide-tooth comb and style the hair while it's wet. Divide the hair into small sections so you won't cause pain. Holding the hair between the roots and where you're combing and keeping it away from the scalp, comb the hair from the ends, gently working your way to the roots.

22. How can I get my child to sit still during hair grooming?

Sit your child in front of the television or pop in a favorite movie or give your child a book to read to you. A snack always works too, or choose a quick and easy hairstyle, like the ones in Chapter 9.

23. Is straightening your hair with a straightening comb damaging?

Yes. It can permanently affect the hair texture. After a period of time, the continuous use of excessive heat can singe and burn your child's hair. This makes the hair weak and often causes the hair to split and break off. Also, the stinky smell released from the hair during pressing is a sure sign of damage. It indicates there is a chemical reaction occurring during the straightening.

24. My baby's hair is thinning around the sides of the head. What should I do?

This is normal. A baby's hair texture is fine, and because they are constantly lying on their backs and sides, babies' fine hair rubs against bed linens and their clothing, which causes some hair thinning. Be patient. As your baby grows, his or her hair will grow back in stronger. Chapter 5 is devoted to newborns.

25. It is normal for a clump of hair to come out of my child's hair after removing a braided style?

We lose about one hundred strands of hair per day. Multiply that figure by the number of days the hair braids have been in, and you'll realize there's not been a terrible amount of hair loss. The hair that usually comes out during the unbraiding process is acceptable. To minimize hair loss, be careful when removing braids and twists. It's important to take your time. Chapter 12 explains the best way to remove braids

26. Does hair grease or oil help the hair to grow?

No it doesn't. Oil assists in the nourishment of hair, but a healthy diet and plenty of water encourages hair to grow. It's important to remember that everyone's hair naturally stops growing when it reaches a certain length and that this varies from person to person.

27. Are rubber bands safe?

No. Tiny strands of hair become tangled in the rubber band, causing serious breakage that can lead to hair loss if continued. Instead, use cloth-covered bands that protect the hair. Some of the covered bands have a small piece of metal on them—be careful! The metal clip against the hair can be just as damaging as a rubber band. Chapter 2 lists hair accessories and ornaments and their use.

28. At what age should I lock my child's hair?

If locking is your and your child's style of choice, I recommend consulting a professional. Remember, locking is a permanent hairstyle. In order to remove locks, they must be cut off. Refer to Chapter 14 for more information about locks.

29. How often should I trim my child's hair?

I recommend trimming your child's hair every four to five months. Remember, there is a difference between cutting and trimming the hair. Trimming the hair means to remove a small amount, less than an inch, all over the head. Cutting the hair is removing an inch or more. I suggest going to a professional for a haircut.

30. How do I remove gum from my child's hair?

Apply ice directly to the hair. Wait for the gum to harden, then carefully break the gum out of your child's hair. Have a talk with your little one and share with them that gum belongs in their mouth only.

31. My daughter cut her hair and it seems almost impossible to cover the spot. What should I do?

Don't panic. It's only hair. It will grow back. Ponytails are a great, simple style that offer plenty of coverage. Chapters 9 and 20 feature styles that may offer you some solutions. If your daughter cut her hair off in the front, then I strongly suggest you take her to a professional.

32. My child swims three to five times a week. How often should I shampoo her hair and what are some of the best style choices?

Chlorine is extremely drying and can have a damaging affect on African-American hair. Daily shampooing is also extremely drying. I suggest that you rinse your daughter's hair with warm water after she swims and add moisture, using natural oils. (See question 20.)

The best hairstyle choices for your daughter's hair are the braids and twists found in Chapter 9. These styles last long and are not ruined by water or chlorine.

33. When I style my child's hair, my parts are always crooked. Are there any tips on making a straight part?

The secret to straight parts is using the point end of the rattail comb.

The rat tail end of the comb helps you slide down the scalp more easily to assist with parting as opposed to using the teeth end. The teeth in the comb may not have the appropriate width to get through the hair depending on the hair's fullness and density. You should use your fingers to separate the hair from the parts you make with the rat tail end of the comb. Practice makes perfect.

34. My daughter came home from school and begged me to put a relaxer in her hair, but I know about the physical and emotional damage relaxers cause. I need some advice.

Read my Introduction and Testimony and have a conversation with your daughter explaining the detriments of chemicals. Help build her self-esteem by constantly reminding her that her hair texture is beautiful just the way it is.

35. Both my son and daughter have locks. A professional stylist started their locks and my children have monthly appointments at the salon. In the summer months, my children are extremely active and prone to getting dirt and debris in their hair while playing. Sometimes I need to clean their hair in between visits to get the dirt out. Is it OK to shampoo their hair and, if so, how do I shampoo their locks?

Yes, you can shampoo the children's hair. Ask your stylist to recommend a shampoo. Sometimes salons sell the shampoos they use on your children. In Chapter 14, there are instructions on how to shampoo locks as well as basic lock maintenance.

36. At the time when I decided to have my daughter's hair locked, I was surprised to find that if I ever wanted to remove the locks, I would have to cut them. Why can't the locks be combed through with a comb?

Locks can't be combed out because of the process locks go through. We shed approximately one hundred strands of hair each day and because there is no combing or brushing of locks, the hair that has been shed doesn't fall or get combed or brushed away. Instead, the shedded hair twists around the lock. If you were to try to comb through the lock you would have a ball of tangled shedded hair that is not attached to the scalp. This is also why locks grow as long as they do.

37. I removed my daughters braid extensions after three months and shampooed her hair. Now I can't comb it through. Her hair is matted all over her head. Do I need to cut all of her hair off?

Don't panic. No, you don't have to cut your child's hair. It can be combed through successfully, but it will take some time and patience. You probably shampooed your child's hair without combing it through thoroughly first. This causes the hair to fuse together and become matted. First rule: You must always comb your child's hair through thoroughly before *you shampoo her hair. This will help when it comes time to style your child's hair.*

Work in small sections and, using your oil and water bottle, spray the area you're working on. Using your fingers, separate the hair. Don't use a comb, which could break your daughter's hair and cause further damage.

Gently pull apart the section of hair you are working with until your daughter's hair is able to be combed. Once you are able to comb the section of hair without ripping the hair, twist or braid the section and clip it out of the way. Repeat this process until the entire head of hair is completed.

19 My Hair

I asked my friend Kim Rodgers, who is a fourth-grade teacher at Benjamin Franklin elementary school in Philadelphia, to ask her students three questions: How would you define your hair? What do you think about your hair? How do others perceive your hair?

The students' responses were interesting. They may reflect some of your own thinking or some of what your child tells you. Hopefully, you will see you and your child are not alone. We hope this book can help you understand what children are thinking and help you feel more committed to putting some of the answers in the book into practice in your life and your child's.

Here are some of the students' honest, funny, and painful responses.

Jamilah

My hair is shoulder length and it is dark brown. In the sunlight, my hair looks reddish brown. My hair is very kinky and curly. When my hair gets wet, it gets very wavy.

If I comb it while it's wet, it doesn't get kinky when it dries. My hair is also thick and grows really slow. When I straighten it, my hair looks really thin.

I think my hair is beautiful. It is easy to do things with it. If I want to braid it or put it in a ponytail, I can do it really quick. I really don't care what people think about my hair. People usually compliment it. Some people say that my hair is nice. I really don't know how people think about my hair because people lie about how you look sometimes.

Latifah

My hair is puffy. Even when I straighten my hair out, it is still puffy. When my hair is wet, it gets really curly and wavy. The root of my hair is wavy but at the tip it's straight. My hair is also really thick and hard to style into a ponytail or bun.

I think my hair is fine the way it is. I feel like my hair describes my individuality. My hair represents my true self and me. If anyone has a problem with my hair then they have a problem.

I think people think I stuck my finger in an electric socket and that's OK with me as long as they see me as a person.

Asha

My hair in the middle is really thick and kinky and around the edges it's thin and soft. My roots are kinky, and it's real soft when it's wet. It's brownish red, and it comes to my neck.

I look at my hair as being real thick but beautiful. I also look at it as being kinky, not nappy.

Really, I don't care about all of the other people's opinions, but I think that other people think I'm not real because I dyed my hair and I get perms. Also I think they think that my hair is nappy. It's not. It's just rough in texture.

Adé

To me, my hair is thick and nappy. My hair reminds me of a pet because it is hard to take care of. My hair is very tangled. I must use a straightening comb to stretch my hair, so I can get a comb through it.

I like my hair, though it is a hard job, and it takes a long time to grow. I think other people look at my hair and get disgusted because it is so nappy. I have had people come to me and say, "Your Afro is bigger than your face."

Renee

Describing my hair is like telling someone about the country I live in. My hair is very curly and thick. That's because I am African American. My hair is brown, shoulder length, and soft.

Actually, I think that my hair is kind of short, very curly, three different colors, soft, and pretty. Some of the ways I take care of my hair are washing, combing, braiding, brushing, and oiling it every time I get a chance.

I think that most of my friends like how soft my hair is and how I keep up with it. But some people think that my hair is too curly. I think they are mad because my hair is longer than theirs.

20 Salon Styles Gallery

Working with the children has been a wonderful experience. I find that children won't always sit still for their parents, but they always sit still for me. The photos included here are, in my opinion, youthful and age-appropriate styles. Keep in mind these same styles can be modified for a more mature look by adding more narrow sections and more part lines, and by omitting childish-looking hair ornaments.

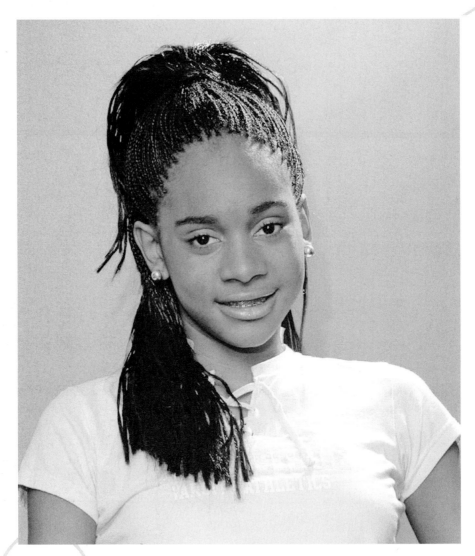

The teenaged Amber wears a more mature style with thin individual braid extensions.

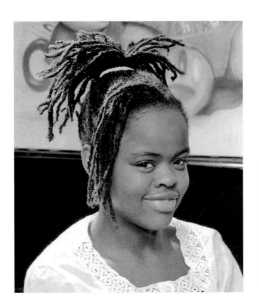

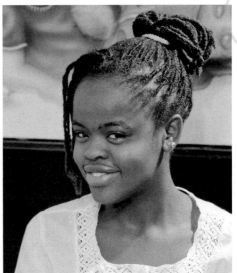

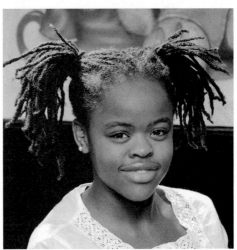

Melissa shows the various ways in which locks can be styled.

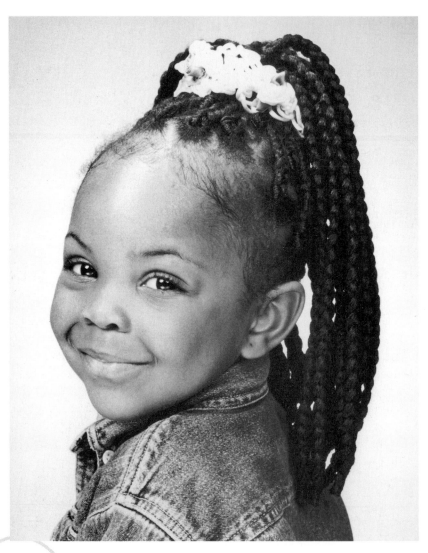

Tatiana sports a Casamas ponytail, where the braids are thick and tightly braided.

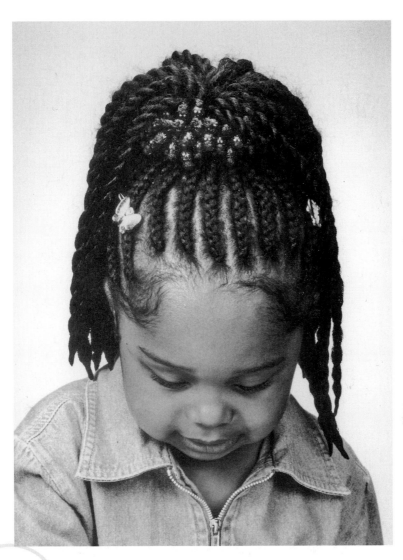

Tycesa has cornrows with a Senegalese ponytail.

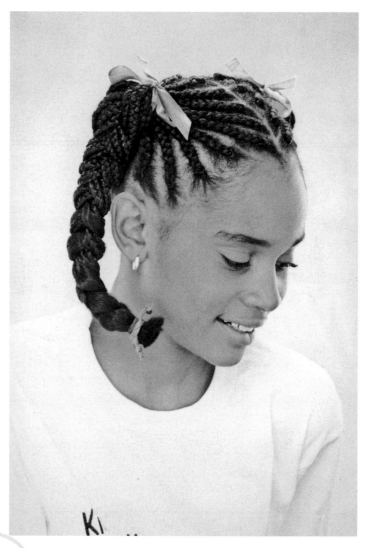

A younger Amber sports cornrows with two braided ponytails.

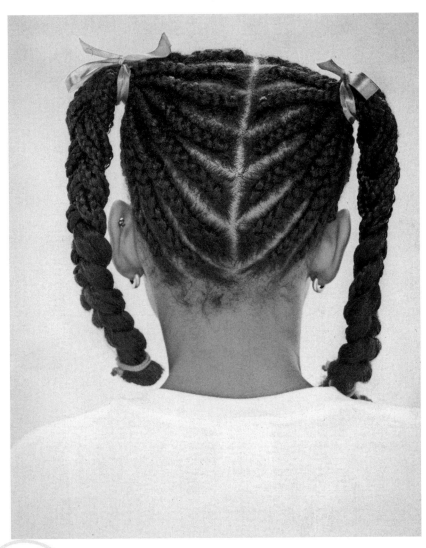

A back view of Amber's cornrows and ponytails.

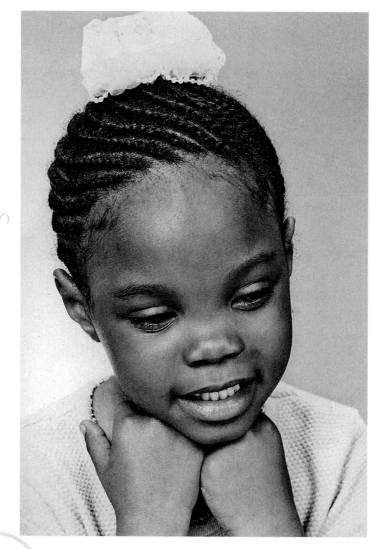

Imani's cornrows were braided diagonally and then set into a bun.

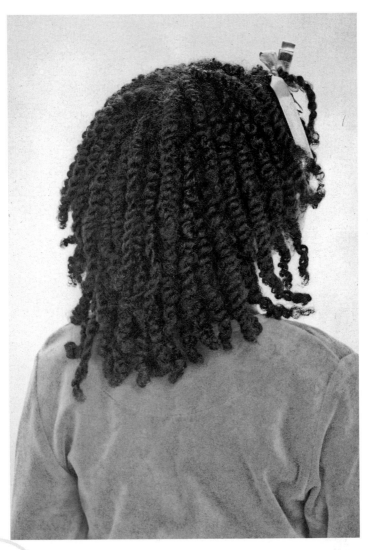

A back view of Simone's two strand twists. (A front view of Simone and her beautiful twists graces the title page of this book.)

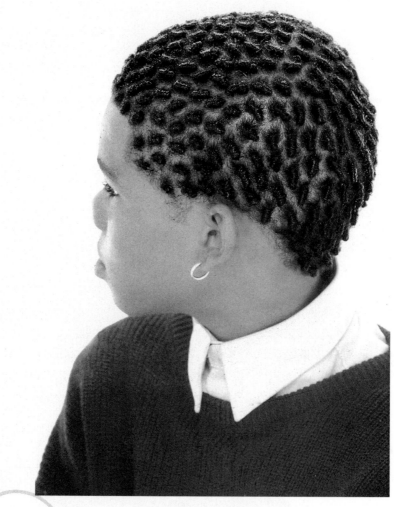

Deione is wearing coils, a style worn by boys.

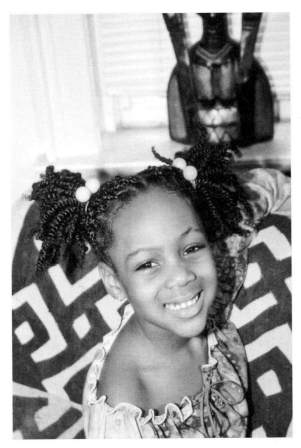

Toni is happy to be wearing
two-strand twists with extensions.

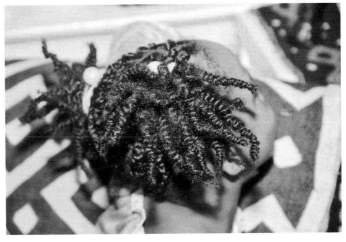

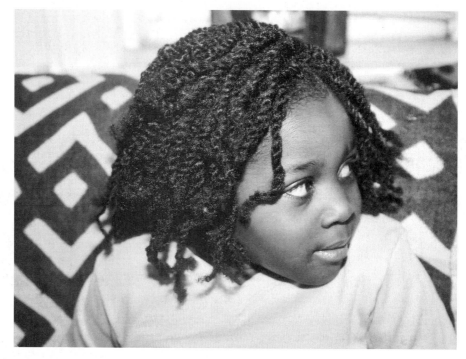

Tyra looks to the side to see who's looking at her two-strand twists.

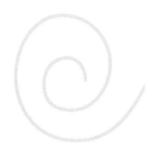

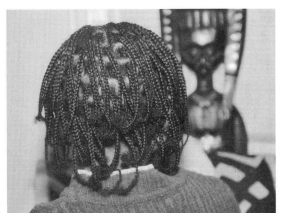

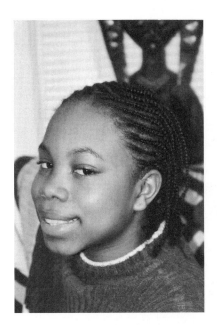

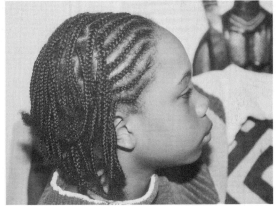

Kadeem sports cornrows with braids hanging loose in the back.

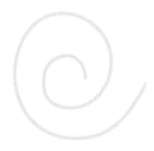

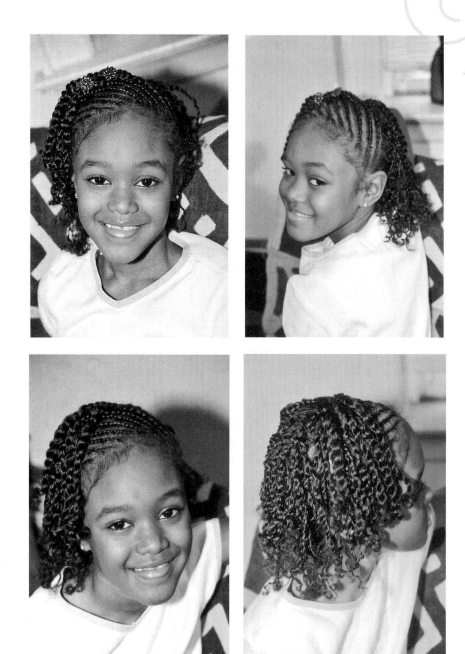

Chynna has been crowned with cornrows and two-strand twists.

Kinki Kreations

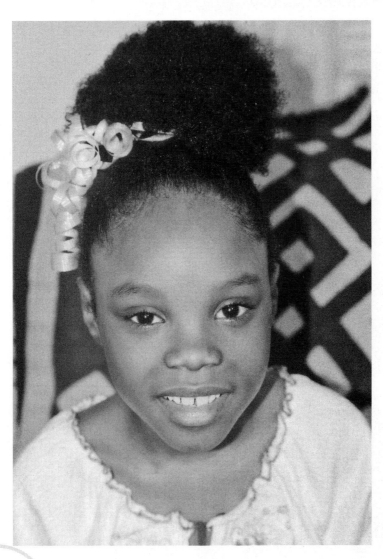

Imani's ponytail gets a jazzy treatment with a spiraling ribbon.

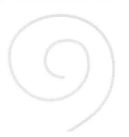

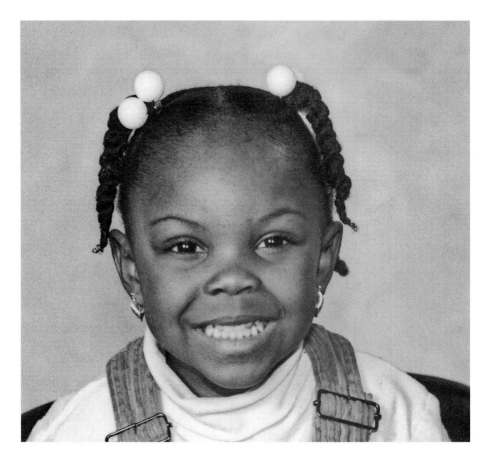

Tatiana has her hair sectioned into four braids with ballies.

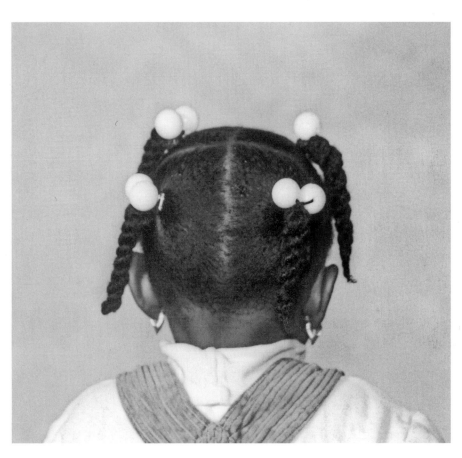

Back view of Tatiana's braids.

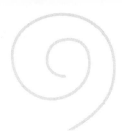

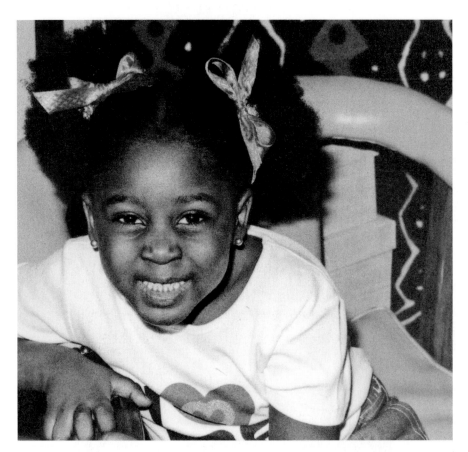

Tyra makes another appearance, this time with ponytail puffs and ribbons.

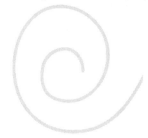

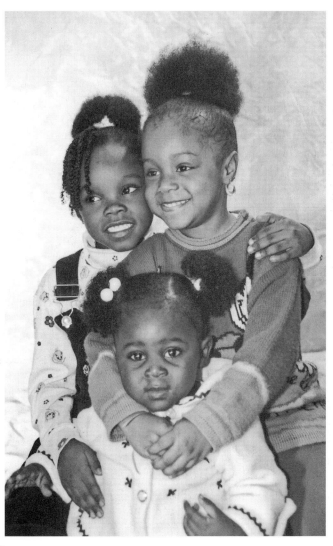

Imani (top left), Briana (top right), and Tyra share the joy of having hairstyles done the natural way.

Glossary

afro—A natural hairstyle in which the hair is shaped into a round, bushy, curly mass.

afro puffs—A hairstyle, characterized by soft "puffs" of natural hair. See Chapter 9.

alopecia—A term that describes a variety of abnormal hair-loss conditions.

alopecia areata—Refers to the sudden or falling out of hair in patches or spots. This condition usually is triggered by trauma to the nervous system.

barrette—An ornament used to adorn the hair often made of plastic and in a variety of shapes and colors.

beads—Small ball-shaped jewelry that can be used to adorn the hair by threading them onto the hair.

bow—A hair ornament that is made from fabric twisted into two or more loops and used for adornment.

braid removal—The act of taking out loose braids, twists, or cornrows.

braid master—One who has technical, artistic, historical, and intellectual authority and expertise in the field of braiding and natural hair care.

braids—Hair that has been divided into three equal sections that are intertwined into a single length of hair. (*Single, box,* and *individual* braids are terms used in the book interchangeably.)

breakage—A condition produced by overprocessing the hair and pulling it too tightly. This is often caused by the unnatural and excessive use of chemicals, dryness, and/or sickness.

brush—A tool composed of bristles set into a handle and used for hair grooming. Boar bristles are used in natural hairbrushes that are best for African-American hair.

Casamas braids—An African hairstyle where the braids are thick in width and tightly braided.

chemical damage—Often devastating external hair loss, scalp burns, and other disorders caused by relaxers, perms, and thermal (hot-iron comb) straightening.

chemicals—Compounds that change the natural texture of the hair, usually causing damage and breakage to the hair.

chlorine—Used as a bleach, oxidizing agent, and disinfectant in water purification; often found in swimming pools. Chlorine can strip the natural oils from your child's scalp.

clips—Hair tools that enclose strands of hair together; often used to keep sections of hair separated and out of the way while combing through after a shampoo and during styling.

clippers—A handheld, motorized device used for cutting hair.

comb—A hair tool, with wide or narrow teeth used for adjusting, detangling, cleaning, or confining hair. The tighter the texture of the hair, the larger and farther apart the teeth should be. This allows for hair to be combed through with minimum stress and hair breakage.

comb out—Separating the hair and leaving it free of tangles.

conditioner—A cream-based (usually liquid) agent that contains vitamins and minerals; it is used to nurture and soften the hair after a shampoo.

consultation—Professional advice from a hairstylist obtained before coming in for a hair appointment. This procedure will ensure clarity on the price, style, length of time the style will last, and any other questions.

cornrows—Three-strand braids interwoven to lay flat on the scalp. They can be designed and sculpted into a variety of patterns with or without extensions.

cradle cap—A common scalp condition found in young babies. It appears as crusty white or yellowish scaly patches on a baby's scalp.

dandruff—Medically known as pityriasis, it is characterized by large scales or flakes on and falling from the scalp.

debris—An accumulation of dirt, lint, and oil that develops on the hair after a period of time.

elasticity—The hair's ability to stretch and return to its original size and shape without breaking.

extensions—Synthetic or human hair, usually in the form of braids and twists, entwined into a hairstyle to add length, fullness, and beauty. Extensions can also be yarn or string.

flaky—The look of debris and dandruff that falls away from the hair and scalp; dandruff flakes are often crusty and usually white or yellowish in color.

flat twists—A braided hairstyle using two strands of hair that lay flat on the scalp. Similar to cornrows.

follicle—The angular, pocketlike depression in the scalp that holds the hair root.

fontanel—The soft spot found at the center of the top of a newborn baby's head.

gels—A clear, semisolid product used to smooth down the hair.

grease—A product used for the hair, very heavy in texture. The main ingredient is petroleum.

grooming—Styling the hair and keeping it neat and clean.

hair—A slender thread outgrowth of the epidermis of the skin and scalp; a cylinder of impacted protein, or keratinized cells.

hair care—Providing and maintaining good health for the hair and scalp.

hair cutting—Removing hair from the head using shears or clippers.

healthy—The condition of being sound in body, mind, or spirit. Free from physical disease or pain.

hot curler—Iron or electric gadget used to curl the hair using heat.

hot iron—Iron or electrical gadget used to straighten the hair using heat.

Kanekalon—A man-made synthetic product, resembling human hair, used to create extended hair.

kiddie perm—Chemicals that remove the natural curl from the hair, straightening it. Usually the same chemicals found in adult perms.

kinky (kinki)—Tightly curled hair.

lock—A natural process of uncut hair that has fused and meshed together.

loose curl—Hair that has a long wave pattern.

lye—A harsh chemical found in perms that is extremely damaging to the hair.

metamorphosis—A transformation that occurs the first or second month after a relaxer has been applied to a child's scalp when the child's relaxed hair hangs limp and dry from the natural growth.

nappy—A negative word used to describe African and African-American hair texture.

peazy—A negative word used to describe African and African-American hair texture.

new growth—Hair that grows naturally from the root of the scalp.

oil—A hair-care product used to add moisture and sheen to the hair.

perm—A hair product used to unnaturally curl the naturally straight texture of the hair. Often used interchangeably with the term *relaxer*, which unnaturally makes kinky hair straight.

petroleum—An oily, flammable paste that is colorless.

ponytail—A hairstyle where the hair is all pulled back away from the face and wrapped in a band to secure it.

rattail comb—A tool with a thin point at one end of the teeth used to style and part the hair and scalp.

relaxer—A hair product that contains harsh chemicals used to unnaturally straighten hair.

ringworm—A disease caused by a fungus (also medically known as *tiena*) that is highly contagious. It can be spread through sharing hair tools.

scalp—The part of the membrane of the human head covered with hair.

sebum—A natural oil produced by the sebaceous glands that adds luster and pliability to the hair and scalp.

shampoo—Detergent used to clean the hair and scalp.

shedding—A natural process that humans undergo, losing approximately one hundred strands of hair per day.

sheen—An appearance of luster and shine.

straighten—Stretching the hair from the original length.

tenderheaded—Pain associated with hair grooming.

tiena—see **ringworm.**

traction alopecia—When the hair is pulled too tight, causing baldness. The hair is literally pulled out of the follicle, taking with it the hair root and the bulb.

transitional denial—When people moving to natural hairstyles become frustrated because they want results quickly. This can result in actions that will impede the process of growing a beautiful head of natural hair.

trim—Removing one to two inches of hair using sheers.

twists—Two strands of hair twisted together.

virgin hair—Hair that has not been altered by chemicals, dyes, heat, or hair straighteners.

wide-tooth comb—Instrument used to comb through hair.

For Further Reading

Bailey, Diane Carol. *Natural Hair Care and Braiding*. New York: Milady Publishing, 1998.

Evans, Nekhena. *Hairlocking: Everything You Need to Know—African, Dread and Nubian Locks*. Brooklyn, N. Y.: New Bein' Press, 1993.

Ferrell, Pamela. *Kids Talk Hair: An Instruction Book for Grown-Ups & Kids*. Washington, D.C.: Cornrows & Co., 1999.

———. *Where Beauty Touches Me*. Washington, D.C.: Cornrows & Co., 1993.

Nappy Hair, illustrated by Joe Cepeda.

hooks, bell. *Happy to Be Nappy*, illustrated by Chris Raschka New York: Hyperion Books, 1999.

Kinard, Talani. *No Lye:* The African American Woman's Guide to Natural Hair Care. New York: St. Martin's Press, 1997.

Mastalia, Francesco, and Alfonse Pagano. *Dreads.* New York: Artisan, 1999.

Morrow, Willie. *400 Years Without a Comb. The Untold Story.* San Diego, Calif.: Morrow's Publishing Research Development, 1990.

Tarpley, Natasha. *I Love My Hair.* New York: Little, Brown and Company: 1998.

Yarbrough, Camille. *Cornrows Illustrated by Carole Byard.* New York: Puffin, 1997.

About
the Author

Master hair braider, locktician, natural hair stylist, and barber, Jena Renee Williams, is a native of Philadelphia, Pennsylvania. Ms. Williams has been a member of several braiding organizations and has been working at her craft since 1987. She is recognized nationally as an innovator and expert in the field.

Ms. Williams is the recipient of several first- and second-place awards. She is a multitalented natural hair-braiding artist whose mastery of more than fifteen techniques and remarkable speed, combined with her signature-styling of the Casamas tight stitch braid, has secured for her a list of impressive clients, which includes talk show hostess and media mogul **Oprah Winfrey;** political activist, educator, and poetess **Sonia Sanchez;** comedian and actress **Thea;** actresses **Kimberly Elise** and **Thandie Newton;** songwriters and vocalists **Rachelle Ferrell** and **Teddy Pendergrass;** and the founder of African-centered festival Odunde, **Lois Fernandez.**

In 1992, Ms. Williams wrote and published the first edition of her quarterly magazine, *Alternative and Solutions.* The photographs and articles served as an instructional guide and manual for other professionals, models, and prospective clients. This effort led to Ms. Williams's organizing and sponsoring annual hair shows, which incorporated dramatic skits, musical performances, and the professional modeling of her most popular and innovative natural hairstyles.

On September 1, 1998, Ms. Williams opened her first salon, Kinki Kreations Braiding Salon, in Philadelphia. She expanded her business on April 1, 2000, adding Kiddie Kreations—Braids and Fades, a salon that caters to children between two and twelve years of age.

Master Braider, Jena Renee Williams, lives by her motto: "Natural hair is a way of life, not a fad!"

Maida Cassandra Odom is a Philadelphia-based journalist, playwright, editor, and teacher. Her mother, Sadie Elizabeth Harvey Odom, taught her that good hair is hair that covers your head.